BREATHE FREE

DISCLAIMER

This book is not intended to treat, diagnose or prescribe. The information contained herein is in no way to be considered as a substitute for your own inner guidance or consultation with a duly licensed health-care professional.

Library of Congress Cataloging-Publication Data

Morningstar, Amadea, 1952-
    -Breathe free : nutritional and herbal care for your respiratory system by Amadea Morningstar & Daniel Gagnon.
    p. cm.
    Includes bibliographical references and index.

    ISBN 0-914955-07-1
    1. Respiratory organs—Diseases—Diet therapy.
    2. Respiratory organs—Diseases—Alternative treatment.
    3. Herbs—Therapeutic use.   4. Dietary supplements—Therapeutic use.   I. Gagnon, Daniel, 1954-
    II. Title.

    RC732.M58 1991
    616.2'004654—dc20   90-24413
                                                                         CIP

Published in 1991 by Lotus Press, P.O. Box 2, Wilmot Wisconsin 53192.

Breathe Free

NUTRITIONAL AND HERBAL CARE
FOR YOUR
RESPIRATORY
SYSTEM

Daniel Gagnon
Amadea Morningstar

Practical Natural Medicine: The Self Help Series

DEDICATION

I dedicate this book to my father, Wilbrod Gagnon. You are the man who has given me the love of wild plants. We would go hunting and return home with a tree for the yard. Thanks. I love you.

Daniel

To the planet and all who live on it.

Amadea

ACKNOWLEDGEMENTS

We wish to thank in alphabetical order:

LaVon Alt
Marge Berra
Lenny Blank
The Bruens
Bill Dean, M.D.
Connie Durand
Emily Esquibel
Trevor Hawkins, M.D.
All the Herbs, Etc. Staff
David Hoffman
Matt Kelly, M.D.
Santosh Krinsky
Patricia Krug
Michael Moore
The Norens
Wes Pittman and the C.S.N. Staff
Mark Sandhaus
Harriet Slavitz
Don Romig, M.D.
Rita Rubin-Gagnon
All of our students, teachers and clients

TABLE OF CONTENTS

Foreword
by David Hoffman

What a joy it was to read this wonderful book. Daniel and Amadea have written an important contribution to the field of holistic health care. Its value lies not only in the therapeutic guidelines given, but also in the way its holistic approach is focused upon this specific but vitally important area of health.

The quality of herbalism and nutrition it contains, embedded in a context of practical considerations, reflect the clinical maturity of these therapists. Especially helpful is the bridging of various healing modalities, exploring as it does herbalism, nutrition, emotional work, body work, and allopathic guidelines. Such well focussed information written by skilled practitioners is often absent from modern herb books. There are some excellent exceptions, but many modern herbals either attempt too much by being all encompassing tomes, or don't go beyond an almost allopathic attachment to specific herbs or favorite formulas for specific diseases. There is a need for many such works examining specific health care issues from the perspective of the phytotherapist in tandem with the knowledge of practitioners of other modalities.

Herbalism has always been the medicine of the people, and still is in most of the world. A responsibility of its practitioners, in such an herbally deprived culture such as ours, is to empower the public with information of the great potentials, and limitations, that herbalism offers. Daniel and Amadea have done this in *Breathe Free*. There is much that herbal medicine can do in the various manifestations of respiratory disease, far more than is often assumed.

I was in practice in West and South Wales for nine years before moving to America, during which time I treated many cases of severe chronic lung problems, from asthma and emphysema to pneumoconiosis (miners' lung) and aspergillosis (farmers' lung). Such industrial 'occupational hazards' were unfortunately all too common in the birthplace of the industrial revolution. Repeatedly I would see herbs, used in an holistic context, facilitate an improvement in these people suffering from what are thought of as degenerative diseases. They were not cured, but experienced marked improvement in the quality of life, and probably length of life as well.

This highlighted an important insight for me. Phytotherapy has most to offer within an integrated health care system when used for the treatment and prevention of chronic problems. There is no denying the achievements of allopathic medicine when it comes to acute infection and emergency procedures. Such advancements should be celebrated but also seen within context. Degenerative disease is now the major killer in the western world, stretching allopathic approaches to their limits. The holistic modalities of healing come into their own here. Our focus should be the whole person and not simply the disease entity.

The authors affirm the role of phytotherapy within the western biomedical model. The move towards holism in healing need *not* mean abandoning the insights of western medicine in favor of the eastern healing traditions. Relevant and effective as they are, we have the opportunity to be part of the transformation that is occurring within western medicine. Acceptance of the bio-medical model as a useful interpretation of the body does not then mean that the analytical and reductionist approach that characterizes modern medicine in the west is the only option. There is a dawning recognition of the possibilities that arise if the bio-medical model is used as a basis for treating the whole person and not simply the disease.

This also leads to the experience of frustration common when people initially explore holistic medicine. There is yet to be written a definitive text on western holistic medicine, a guide that clearly illuminates these new and exciting perspectives. There is a veritable maelstrom of activity amongst holistic practitioners, exploring and applying new ideas but it is still in the early days.

For some this is just too frustrating, leading to an abandonment of the endeavor or a turning to one of the oriental systems. For others this is a very exciting time to be involved in medicine. The unclarity of the situation is one aspect of a flowering of new ideas. There is no comprehensive text book because the ideas have not reached the stage where they can be written in stone. It is a time of flux, where many new insights are being obtained and old ideas are being reassessed and discarded or embraced anew.

Breathe Free is an excellent example of the harvest of ideas our culture is reaping from those exploring holism. Herbs fit perfectly within a holistic context, but are not in themselves holistic. In the hands of a skilled holistic practitioner, who has an understanding of both the plant and the person, phytotherapy can facilitate profound healing and 'wellness'. *Breathe Free* is a book that applies herbs and nutrition in this holistic way. As a teacher of future phytotherapists, this book helps me 'Breath Easy' knowing that western herbalism is being given this quality of attention and development.

The authors are to be congratulated on their reintroduction of 'forgotten' medicinal plants such as Stillingia, Wild Indigo and Quassia. I hope that in future volumes in this series they mention Balmony, Fringetree, Life Root, and the wealth of other North American medicinals that have been lost sight of in this country but are still used extensively in Europe. I also greatly appreciate their affirming the value of the less 'glamorous' healing plants such as Nettles! Herbs don't have to be imported or expensive to be good medicine.

Profound developments are occurring within herbalism throughout the World. The field of herbal medicine, now known as phytotherapy in Europe, is being rediscovered by all involved in health care. This includes, of course, both public and professionals! This dispersal of the collective amnesia about herbal medicine has a number of factors underlying it. To mention just a few:

- because it works!
- because it is a lot less expensive
- because it is environmentally sound

Whilst there is not the space here to explore these in depth, the last is too important to leave alone. From the perspectives of an eco-activist, it can be argued that many health issues are internalizations of cultural, ecological and planetary dis-ease. The psychoanalysts attention on alienation is possibly a subset of our species alienation from nature. Herbalism has a role to play in bridging this separation. The medieval herbalist, Hildegard Von Bingan, talks of 'viriditas', the Greening power. The healing offered so abundantly and freely by the plant kingdom is indeed a greening of the human condition, pointing to the reality of a new springtime. Humanity is awakening and finally becoming present within the biosphere, vibrantly alive, eyes wide open with hearts that feel the love of the Whales and the Redwoods, minds revivified, filled with visions of a healed world and ready for the challenges ahead.

This unprecedented but timely renaissance, as Dr. Paul Lee has called it, highlights the responsibility of professional herbalists to communicate their skills and knowledge in a way that is relevant to the needs of people now. Daniel and Amadea have done this. Thank you both.

David Hoffman
The apple orchards of West Sonoma County, California
November, 1990

INTRODUCTION: ABOUT THIS BOOK

Our experience as health care practitioners and educators spans a combined total of twenty-seven years. During this time we have observed and listened with respect, attention and care to the people with whom we have worked. What we learned in this way has strongly influenced the format and underlying philosophy of this book.

Like many other health care practitioners, we discovered that the body, mind and feelings all influence health and healing, in an inter-related way. We also have observed that the more people take charge of their own health care programs, the more effective are the results. So our general approach has become one which honors the profound influence of feelings, mind and body working together in healing. It supports the self-empowerment of our clients.

Our approach in writing this book reflects the perspective we use in our practices. For the mind, we explain what is going on in each disorder process in the *Definition, Description* and *Biological Overview* sections of each chapter.

Physicians will notice that in a book framed chiefly (although not exclusively) for the layperson, we do not observe the technical distinction between "signs" and "symptoms." Medical terms have been kept to a minimum, and the general reader will find such words defined in the Glossary at the back of the book.

This is followed by *Emotional Information*, based upon our experience with each disorder. This material is by no means offered as the last word on the subject. Rather, it is intended to spur the reader on the path of self-discovery toward a recognition of the emotional stresses and struggles that ask for attention and healing. Exploring this process can benefit not only the mind and feeling heart, but the physical body as well.

In *Guidelines for Action*, priorities are set: what measures should be taken, and in what order, to most effectively restore health.

Therapeutic Recommendations include sections on *Foods, Botanicals* and *Supplements*. In our experience the three are most effective when used together, offering optimal support. They may, of course, be used separately. For example, if you have no access to herbs and supplements you still can use foods as a healing tool.

Basis of Therapeutics was born of our frustration with many source books which give excellent lists of healing tools—herbs, vitamins, foods—but which neglect to explain why they are recommended and how they work. *Basis of Therapeutics* does just that. This information is in process, and we have offered the most up-to-date information with which we are familiar. We anticipate revisions as the bank of knowledge about alternative healing energetics and methods grows.

Prevention and Healing gives a long-term overview on the wellness process. This is the section you will want to consult first if the illness threatens to recur, or if you have concerns that it could become chronic. Here we make suggestions for specific preventive and healing regimens: what measures to use or to avoid.

The closing section, *Visualization*, invites participation in an experiential process designed to involve the emotions, body and mind in their own deeper healing. We use these processes in our private practices to access the inner healing forces, encouraging the body to relax, let go,and move into an affirmative state of healing. It may be helpful to have a friend slowly and gently read this section to you. Or tape it for yourself, reading at a relaxed pace. You may find that our suggestions here stimulate other images of healing specific to you. Trust their power and allow the process to unfold.

Orthodox medicine tells us that either we are healthy or sick. If no definable disease is found, often there is no relief for a discomfort that may be very real. Or, if we are found to be sick, for example with pneumonia, the doctor prescribes antibiotics and hopes that the body eventually will rebalance itself. In both cases, herbs and nutrition can offer substantial support to help regain that balance with less stress or cost to the body.

In our view, disease is not simply an enemy to be eradicated without a second thought. It can be the ally that shows us a new perspective, an opportunity toward change. Rightly and fully understood, it can open doors to new and healthier ways of being.

It is our hope that this book, too, will open doors to a new perspective which supports the body and the earth in much needed healing. We welcome your response to the information presented here. All of our support and participation are vital at this time to create the sorely needed healing of our planet and us all.

Amadea Morningstar & Daniel Gagnon
Santa Fe, New Mexico, Summer 1991

ABOUT HERBS

When taking herbs, please be aware of the following:

1. If you are taking herbs for a specific condition and are not getting better or are getting worse, promptly consult with a doctor or a qualified herbalist. All therapies, including herbal therapy, have limits.

2. In an acute situation, it is best to take a smaller amount of the herb and to take it more often. If a normal dosage is 30 drops every three hours, taking five drops every half hour will insure that the extract is always in the bloodstream. It is best to first take a full dose (i.e., 30 drops), then five drops every half hour.

3. In a chronic situation, patience is necessary. In such cases treatment is aimed at the deficient organ or tissue, which often responds slowly. Adequate amounts of the extract must be taken on a regular basis and for a sustained period of time to effect a change. Full results may take weeks. For chronic diseases (e.g., emphysema), it is sometimes best to take the extract for one month, stop for two weeks, and repeat.

Very rarely are herbs used to kill microbes directly. In this regard, herbs function differently from most synthetic drugs. Herbs work by strengthening and stimulating body systems. They support the body's effort to neutralize toxins and foreign matters, and decrease the physical stress of disease. For these reasons herbs tend to work more slowly than drugs and yet are more effective in preventing recurrences and/or further damage from the illness.

As an example, antibiotics may be used effectively when the illness is in an active crisis stage. Herbs are used (most effectively) at the first signs of disease before conditions become extreme, though they can usually be used as support even in these cases. Awareness and self-responsibility are key concepts here.

4. When using extracts, always put the dose in four to

eight ounces of liquid. This will increase its dispersion and absorption into the body. The liquid may be water, juice or herbal teas. Beverages that contain caffeine, such as coffee, tea and colas, impede the absorption of botanical constituents.

5. Many herbs are unstable once they have been ground. This applies to golden seal, echinacea and osha, for example. Encapsulated herbs, since they are ground, are unstable. It is recommended that you use only prepared liquid herbal extracts made from freshly ground herbs, fresh herbs or whole herbs that you then freshly grind yourself.

6. Liquid herbal extracts permit custom tailoring of the dosage. In order to meet their individual therapeutic requirements, thin and older people may reduce the dosage by a few drops, while heavier people can use a few more drops.

7. Good quality extracts are made with a high percentage of alcohol (40 to 95 percent). Persons who should not use alcohol may boil some water, pour it into a cup, add as many drops of herbal extracts as desired, and let it sit for seven to ten minutes. Approximately 95 percent of the alcohol will evaporate.

8. The formulas in this book have been composed in a specific way. The milder herbs which may be taken in larger quantities are listed first, followed by the stronger herbs which should be taken in smaller quantities. If you decide to put your own formulas together, remember that you can safely use more of the milder (first listed) herbs and should limit the use of the more potent (listed last) ones.

9. *Certain herbs, notably the following, should be used with caution:*
• Ma Huang if taken in excessive amounts may produce insomnia, anxiety, restlessness, loss of appetite, nausea, muscular weakness and tremors. In small amounts it acts as an effective bronchial dilator.

• Blood Root in excessive doses (from 8 to 20 drops) acts as a gastric irritant. It produces burning pains in areas from the mouth to the stomach, dilated pupils, nausea, anxiety, coldness of the extremities and a slowed pulse. In very small amounts, it activates blood circulation in the lungs.

• Poke Root in overdose (½ ounce of the root) may produce vomiting, diarrhea, drowsiness, vertigo, tingling of the whole body, dimness of vision, cold skin, feeble pulse, convulsion and possibly coma. In small amounts, it acts as an excellent immune system stimulant.

• Lobelia in excessive amounts may produce depression, nausea, cold sweats, progressive vomiting, tremors, convulsions, coma and death. In small amounts it is a powerful respiratory stimulant.

ABOUT SUPPLEMENTS

Supplements are offered throughout this book as one option in healing. Due to modern agricultural and food preparation practices, our foods have become notably depleted in many nutrients. This is particularly true of the essential trace minerals usually preserved through organic composting methods— chromium, zinc, selenium, manganese, and magnesium, to name a few. As another example, when whole wheat is refined to white flour it loses approximately 90 per cent of its vitamin E. It has been estimated that at the turn of this century in America, the average daily intake of vitamin E was 160 I.U.'s per person. Now it is less than 60 I.U.'s, primarily because of this shift away from whole grains. While many Americans have begun to pursue healthier nutrition practices in recent years, the deficits from years of eating "non-whole" foods can be long-lasting. Supplements provide one fairly short-term means (i.e., one to two years or less) for most people to replenish their nutritional stores.

Nutritional supplements are not indicated for everyone. Some people will choose to get all of their nourishment from whole foods. Appendix C p.133 provides information about the richest, commonly available food sources of the various essential nutrients.

Some people who may wish to use supplements may find that some vitamins or minerals cause them indigestion, rash, or other discomforts. For this reason, it is best to begin to add supplements one at a time (i.e., one per day) at the lowest recommended dose. If you continue to be confronted with side effects, it is advisable to stop the supplements for a short time and to consult an experienced health care practitioner.

It is important to follow the therapeutic recommendations as to *when* to take supplements as these recommendations are designed for maximal absorption and ease of digestion.

Also carefully observe the suggested dosages since, like other concentrated substances, nutritional supplements can be toxic. This is especially true of vitamins A and D. A normal daily dose for adults is 5,000-10,000 I.U. of vitamin A and 400 I.U. of vitamin D. Many multiples include amounts far in excess of this in the daily dose, which can produce ill effects. Vitamin A as beta-carotene usually can be tolerated in substantially larger amounts; for most people 25,000 I.U. per day for a long period would be quite safe.

If you are taking digitalis for your heart, no extra vitamin E (above 100 I.U. per day) should be taken without your physician's specific recommendation. If you have high blood pressure, vitamin E should be taken in smaller doses than is recommended in most of this text. High doses of vitamin E (equivalent to 800 I.U. per day or more) can cause a transient but potentially dangerous increase in blood pressure. This can be avoided by slowly increasing vitamin E doses from 200 I.U. per day in the first week of taking it to 400 I.U. per day in the second week, to 600 I.U. per day in the third week. In one month you can be safely taking the 800 I.U. dose, which can have a strengthening effect on both heart and lungs. If you have any questions about this, please consult a trusted health care practitioner/nutritionist.

Previously it was assumed that water-soluble vitamins (the B complex and vitamin C) were non-toxic, as they are readily excreted in the urine. In the past three decades, unusually high doses of these vitamins have been taken and it is becoming clear that one can get too much of a water-soluble nutrient. The most common side effect of excess vitamin C is diarrhea, which usually clears when the vitamin is stopped. In rare cases, excess vitamin C has been reported to exacerbate or create kidney stones in genetically susceptible individuals. This is usually prevented with an adequate intake of fluids (and magnesium in some cases). Doses of vitamin B_6 (pyridoxine) are now generally kept to under 200 mg. per day. Long-term intake at above 200 mg. per day has been associated with peripheral and permanent nerve damage.

Most people taking 50,000 I.U. of vitamin A per day for two weeks or longer could react with such symptoms of acute toxicity as hair loss, fatigue, irritability and bone pain. Taken over a long period, 1,000 I.U. of vitamin D per day can cause similar symptoms.

Some supplements may be appropriate for you where others are not. The *Basis of Therapeutics* section in each chapter gives information which you can use to help you make choices about each nutrient.

Supplements come in a variety of forms. If you have difficulty swallowing, chewables, lozenges or liquid tonics will be most useful. If you are subject to various kinds of "dryness"—for example, of the skin, hair or bowels—oilier capsules will probably be more appropriate than large dry tablets. If you have a history of food sensitivity, the hypo-allergenic brands have the most to offer you. If you have the classic "cast-iron" stomach, probably most forms will suit you if they are taken at the appropriate times. This is usually after meals or at bedtime. The amino acids—L-glutamine, L-cysteine,—are exceptions to this rule. They are best absorbed if taken 15 minutes before a meal.

Special WARNING note for pregnant women and for young children. Doses should be kept conservatively small. Please note the differences in Therapeutic Recommendations for children and for adults. In pregnancy it is especially important to restrict your supplemental intake of vitamin A to 20,000 I.U. per day or *less.* Larger doses can cause birth defects. Vitamin E intake should be kept to 200 I.U. per day or less, for maximal placental balance. In pregnancy, vitamin C intake should be kept to 1,000 mg. per day or less, as high doses may cause a vitamin C dependent scurvy in new-born infants withdrawn from this rich supply. Conversely, it is important in pregnancy to get *more* folic acid than you would normally need (800-1200 mcg. per day), in order to promote healthy growth of the fetus and prevent neural tube defects.

ABOUT OUR ENVIRONMENT

It's going fast. The earth is the body on which we live. How the earth feels affects how we feel, subtly or grossly. If the air you breathe is dirty, you can count on the inside of your lungs being dirty as well.

Trees are the lungs of our environment. They clear the air and balance the earth's carbon dioxide to oxygen ratio. Without them, the "greenhouse effect" grows. And millions of trees die each day.

Like an atmospheric membrane, the ozone layer shields and protects our globe from the radiation ever present in space. Without trees and a healthy intact ozone, concern for individual health becomes almost ludicrous. Many races and many species are ailing or already lost. The number of peculiar microbes harbored by species, such as the proliferation of canine distemper virus in dolphins in the North Sea, is bizarre yet now commonplace. As the human race we risk our own extinction through a system of demands and expectations unrealistic for our planet or our long-term survival.

Land fills represent congested areas deep within the bowels of the earth. In these garbage-filled regions covering many square miles of planet, air cannot be exchanged, normal mineral exchanges do not occur, and light does not penetrate. A hot dog disposed of 15 years before can be found intact. This is not breakdown and elimination of wastes, but simply storage of them. In many areas, especially in nuclear waste dumps, the breakdown which does manage to occur creates more toxic and explosive by-products than the original wastes (such as those in Hanford, Washington). Our "bowels" are having serious problems.

Much has been written about how best to address this disease on a personal, community and planetary level. Personally we can routinely ask ourselves, as our hand hovers over the garbage can, "Does this need to be put in cold storage for decades or can it be recycled or used somewhere else in our homes?'' Or at the mall, ''Do I really need this product or have I got something already which works nearly as well? How much can I contribute to cleansing, clearing and elimination now?''

If there is an area which has been disturbing you or your health, think about acting on it now. What is bothering you? And what can you do about it?

ANATOMY AND PHYSIOLOGY

For ready reference, here is a brief overview of the structure and function of the respiratory system. The books cited in the bibliography provide more detailed information for the interested reader.

RESPIRATORY SYSTEM

UPPER RESPIRATORY TRACT

Functions:

Nose
—directs air into the respiratory system
—hairs stop entrance of large particles into the respiratory system

Nasal Cavity
—conducts, warms and humidifies air
—mucus traps smaller particles and bacteria

Sinuses
—act as a resonance chamber enhancing the quality of the voice

Pharynx
(also known as Throat)
—directs food to the stomach and air to the lungs
—aids in sound/speech production

Larynx
(also known as Voice Box)
—houses vocal cords
—directs air to the lungs
—its mucus filters air

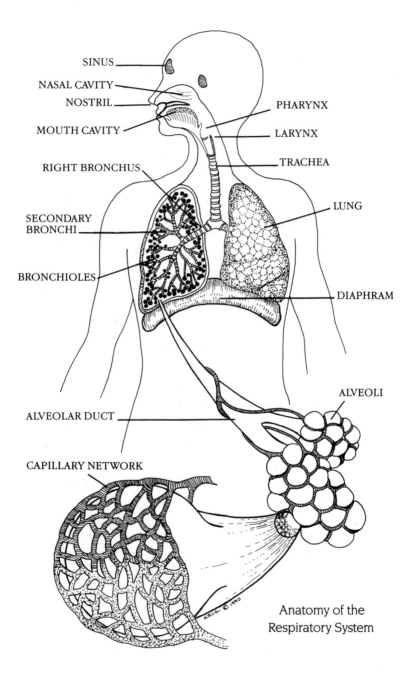

SINUS

NASAL CAVITY

NOSTRIL

MOUTH CAVITY

PHARYNX

LARYNX

TRACHEA

RIGHT BRONCHUS

LUNG

SECONDARY BRONCHI

BRONCHIOLES

DIAPHRAM

ALVEOLI

ALVEOLAR DUCT

CAPILLARY NETWORK

Anatomy of the Respiratory System

Trachea   —directs and filters air
Bronchial Tree
Lungs:
   Alveolar Walls   —receives oxygen and expels
   Blood Vessels   carbon dioxide and other gases
   Connective Tissue
   Nerves
   Lymphatic Vessels

Fascinating Facts

   Did you know that . . .
   —the right lung is larger than the left one and has 3 lobes
    while the left one has only 2!
   —by the time the air inhaled through the nose reaches
    the lower trachea it is within 2-3 degrees of the body's
    temperature and within 2-3 per cent of full saturation
    of water vapor!
   —one side of the sinuses is engorged with blood for one
    hour and then it's the other side's turn. This explains
    why you can breathe better from one nostril at a given
    moment, after which the other seems to work better!
   —there are 300 million alveoli. If all of these were open
    and laid flat, they would cover an area of 25 x 30 feet
    or 750 square feet, roughly the size of a tennis court!
   —there is only ¼ to ½ cup (2 to 4½ ounces) of blood
    being oxygenated in the lungs at any given time.
    Imagine this small amount of blood thinly covering an
    entire tennis court!
   —the capillaries on the surface of the alveoli are so small
    that the red blood cells can only pass through them in
    single file!
   —when air is inspired it contains 21 per cent oxygen and
    .04 per cent carbon dioxide. Expired air contains
    about 16 per cent oxygen (a 20 per cent decrease) and
    about 3.6 per cent carbon dioxide (a 1000 percent

increase)!

— healthy lungs use only 2-3 per cent of the body's total energy during normal quiet respiration. But when a lung is diseased, up to 33 percent of the body's energy may be expended for respiration alone!

— in an average day a person takes about 12 breaths a minute or 17,280 breaths a day.

Things to Remember when Caring for Your Respiratory System

1. If you're not getting better in 3 to 5 days or actually are getting worse, see a doctor or other knowledgeable health care practitioner.

2. Productive coughing (i.e., mucus coming up) should not be suppressed. A dry irritating cough which prevents sleep or is exhausting you can be suppressed.

3. Fever is useful and helps fight off infection. It is only a danger if it exceeds 104° for a prolonged period of time. Otherwise, ensure adequate fluids and electrolytes replacement (see Healing Broth, p. 132) and use cold soaks in place of Tylenol™ or aspirin.

4. Postural drainage and percussion to the back helps break up congestion and mucus.

5. Heat to the chest will also break up lung congestion. This includes hot packs, Tiger Balm™, heating pads, or Vicks VapoRub™.

THE COMMON COLD/ INFLUENZA

DEFINITION

Sometimes called the flu, the common cold is a viral infection of the mucous membranes of the nasal passages and trachea.

Note: Antibiotics are *not* effective in treating the common cold as they kill only bacteria. They are useful only in treating and preventing secondary bacterial infections.

DESCRIPTION

Symptoms include general malaise, muscle and joint aches, headache, mucus discharge from the nose, post-nasal drip, sneezing, scratchy throat, cough, chills and irritability. Fever usually is low and intermittent. Many respiratory viruses may initiate the common cold, against which the body builds only temporary immunity.

Untreated flu can spread to the lungs. In such cases, flu may lead to severe pneumonia. *High risk groups are the elderly, children, women in late pregnancy and persons with cardiac or pulmonary disease. People with immunosuppressive diseases and those who use immunosuppressive medications also are at risk. If you are in one of these categories, or are caring for someone who is, extra TLC and preventative care are needed.*

Prompt and sustained treatment of the common cold is very important, since it can cause or aggravate most of the other diseases covered in this book.

BIOLOGICAL OVERVIEW

Louis Pasteur, who for many years searched for microorganisms as the cause of disease, noticed that in many cases microorganisms precipitated an illness only if certain environmental factors also were present. *It is the condition of the host and not the virus or bacteria that is the critical factor.* People who are tired, under stress, not exercising sufficiently and/or are malnourished are more susceptible to colds than those who lead a healthy life. The common cold is a signal to slow down and to take care of yourself.

Once the cold is there, it is best to work with it, to rest and sweat it out.

As early as 100 B.C., Parmenides recorded this observation: "Give me a chance to create a fever and I will cure any disease." A fever provides an excellent means to work with the immune system. German research in the 1950s showed that the body uses fever to activate white blood cells, speed up metabolism and slow down the growth of invading viruses or bacteria.

Fever also stimulates the eliminative and detoxifying capacities of the skin. Therefore it is important not to suppress a moderate fever (99° to 102°F) with aspirin or similar drugs, as they inhibit the body's elimination channels. In addition, when there is little or no elevation of temperature, aspirin offers little symptomatic relief. Furthermore, aspirin has been shown to increase the shedding of viruses during the contagious stage of the flu, thereby increasing the possibility of infecting those around you.

Note: An alternative to aspirin for children or pregnant women is Oscillococcinum™, a homeopathic remedy. Cold packs can also be used to bring down fevers above 102°F, and should be used promptly to prevent tissue damage especially in children.

EMOTIONAL INFORMATION

Colds and flu often arise when we are doing more than we can comfortably handle. The body creates this (welcome or unwelcome) respite for itself in the midst of overexertion. Sometimes colds, especially thick congested head colds, can be an indicator of confusion. Often, simply giving yourself the time and rest it takes to heal the cold, provides the space within your mind and heart to clear up what may be confusing you. Sometimes there is a tendency to feel victimized or put upon by the flu, and this can be addressed. Take it easy on yourself.

GUIDELINES FOR ACTION

1. Rest.
2. Stimulate the immune system.
3. Alkalize the whole body.
4. Provide ample hydration and electrolytes.
5. Activate eliminative processes (e.g., sweating).
6. Strengthen the areas under stress (e.g., nose and throat).

THERAPEUTIC RECOMMENDATIONS
FOODS

Foods which are alkalizing should be used in a ratio of at least 4:1 to foods which are acidifying. Alkalizing foods are those which, when digested and metabolized, produce an alkaline residue or ash in the body. These foods include almost all vegetables and fruits (except cranberries and prunes). Plenty of fresh pure water and fresh fruit or vegetable juices are especially useful. Acidifying foods tend to aggravate or prolong common colds and should be used minimally or avoided. Strongly acidifying foods include alcohol, sugar, red meat, concentrated proteins, coffee and sweets.

Dairy foods such as milk, cheese and ice cream are best avoided as they can exacerbate congestion. Whole grains are neutral in charge (neither strongly positive nor negative) and may be used in moderation. It is best to eat to appetite. The healing broth (see p. 132), as well as other clear vegetable soups, is excellent and alkalizing.

BASIS OF THERAPEUTICS

Fruits and vegetables have been prescribed for centuries as a traditional cure for colds and flu. Their alkalizing effect is one likely reason for their effectiveness. A healthy human body has a slightly negative charge, i.e., is mildly alkaline. Viruses, the carriers of flu, are also slightly negatively charged. Thus, since like charges repel, a normally healthy negatively charged body will repel most viruses in its environment. According to one hypothesis, bodies under stress, and those taking in large amounts of alcohol, sweets, or meat, become more positively charged (acidic), thereby attracting viruses. Fruits and vegetables, being rich sources of vitamins and electrolytes, are particularly well-suited to alkalize the system.

BOTANICALS

SWEAT TEA

Yarrow	1 part	Steep ½ ounce of this mixture in 1 pint hot water for 20 minutes. Drink 1 or 2 cups before and during a hot bath.
Elder Blossoms	1 part	
Boneset	1 part	

Echinacea	3 parts	Take as a capsule or tablet. Take 2 tablets every 4 hours during the infection.
Garlic	2 parts	
Osha	2 parts	
Cayenne	1 part	

IMMUNE SYSTEM TONIC

Echinacea	6 parts	As a preventative take 20-30 drops 2-4 times a day. During infection take up to 45 drops every hour.
Osha	2 parts	
Astragalus	2 parts	
Calendula (in fresh form only	1 part	

Echinacea Extract: Take 30-80 drops every hour during the infection.

"Hot brew for colds": two or three cinnamon sticks, 1 inch of fresh ginger and 2 tablespoons of hibiscus flowers steeped in 1 quart of boiled water. This a helpful tea for both children and adults. It is warming and speeds healing, and may be mixed with orange juice or honey to taste.

> Note: During pregnancy, echinacea, garlic, and a combination of cinnamon, ginger and hibiscus may be taken. Avoid the other herbs.

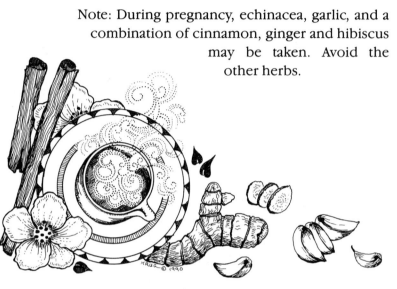

BASIS OF THERAPEUTICS

Yarrow: Helps break dry fevers. Stimulates excretion of waste products and pyrogens through sweating.

Elder Blossoms: Stimulates sweating. Works with the fever. Breaks up nasal congestion caused by the flu.

Boneset: Relieves deep-seated bone and joint pains caused by common cold viruses. Also relieves scratchy throat and coughs.

Echinacea: Has an interferon-like action against viruses. Stimulates T-cells. Enhances all functions of the immune system.

Garlic: Helps prevent secondary respiratory infections. Slows the spreading of viruses by preventing clumping of lymphocytes.

Osha: Stimulates resistance to viruses. Reduces inflammation of the throat. Increases sweating in hot feverish states.

Cayenne: Increases blood flow through stressed tissues. Acts as a catalyst for the other herbs.

Astragalus: Deep immune system stimulant. Will build excellent resistance and improve immune function.

Calendula: Must be used in fresh or fresh freeze-dried forms. Dried will not work. Works similarly to Echinacea. Supports the immune system in its functions.

SUPPLEMENTS

Beta-carotene—30,000-100,000 I.U. per day total, taken after meals for no more than 5 days. See the warning note in ABOUT SUPPLEMENTS, p. 8.

Zinc lozenges—15 mg. 5 times per day for first 5 days; 3 times per day thereafter.

Buffered vitamin C—1,000-10,000 mg. per day, up to 1,000 mg. per hour.

A Good Multiple Vitamin and Mineral Formula (see p. 146).

Garlic—1 capsule, 3-5 times per day with meals.

BASIS OF THERAPEUTICS

Beta-carotene (vitamin A): Stimulates white blood cell activity and localized immune defenses. It is a potent strengthener of the immune system against flus, and as effective or more so for many people than vitamin C.

Zinc (in lozenge form): Promotes production of T-cell and T-helper cells, vital immune defenders. Zinc releases vitamin A from the liver. It can significantly reduce severity and duration of the common cold.

Buffered vitamin C: The popular cold preventive, though few studies have been able to support this widespread claim. Many of our clients report that vitamin C is helpful.

This supportive action may derive from its ability to stimulate interferon production in white blood cells. Interferon, a natural viral antagonist, then attacks the flu virus. However, the exact mechanism of vitamin C's action in fighting the common cold is not yet fully understood.

A Good Multiple Vitamin and Mineral Formula: Supports a coordinated immune defense and whole body healing.

Garlic: see BASIS OF THERAPEUTICS, p. 21.

PREVENTION AND HEALING

At the very first signs of a cold, it is suggested that copious amounts of echinacea extract be taken: 40 to 80 drops every hour until you feel well. To combat the cold, up to 100,000 units daily of vitamin A in the form of beta-carotene may be taken for up to 5 days *except in pregnancy or if you are trying to conceive.* See ABOUT SUPPLEMENTS, p. 9. Zinc lozenges can be sucked if there is any throat involvement. 3-10 grams of vitamin C also are recommended.

Liquids: Drink as much as 3 quarts of fluids per day.

Hot bath: Taking a hot bath at the onset of a cold helps to stimulate the body's defenses. It also increases elimination of toxins through the skin. Drink Sweat Tea (see p. 20) before and during the bath. Stay in water as warm as you can stand for at least 15 minutes. Then dry yourself and go directly to bed. You will continue to sweat. Rest. Relax.

Humidifier: A humidifier can prevent the recurrence of infections caused by poorly hydrated mucous membranes.

Recurrent colds indicate an overly acidic system, excessive stress, a poorly functioning immune system, or all of the above. Review all the nutrients needed for a healthy immune system, including iron, selenium, vitamins C and A, zinc, vitamin B complex and pantothenic acid. Are you getting ample amounts of these? Or is your susceptibility primarily a matter of not enough sleep, too much exertion, and too many acidifying substances in your diet? If it is any of the latter, correcting these imbalances and utilizing in smaller quantities the therapeutic herbs prescribed here to rebuild your immune system is suggested. It also should be understood that drugs and alcohol are potent inhibitors of the immune system.

Exercise is a powerful stimulant for a sluggish lymphatic system. Acupuncture can be a helpful support for a flagging immune system, when combined with proper diet, herbs and activity.

VISUALIZATION

There is nothing you need to do but rest. Your body can take care of this infection, and it will. Give it the time and space it needs to heal. You can imagine that it is a vast and healthy landscape. A small congested area is about to be cleansed gently and directly.

ALLERGIC RHINITIS: HAY FEVER

DEFINITION

Seasonal hay fever and chronic inflammation of the nose, throat and sinuses are forms of allergic rhinitis. This inflammation is induced by external irritants.

DESCRIPTION

Symptoms of allergic rhinitis include inflammation; watery, irritated eyes; drippy nose; post-nasal drip; sneezing or coughing attacks; and itchy eyes and nose. An irritated or sore throat may develop. Frontal headaches, loss of appetite, nausea, asthmatic symptoms and insomnia also may be present.

Allergic rhinitis is classified into two categories:

a) Seasonal hay fever is caused by wind-borne pollens. Spring hay fever usually is set off by tree pollen (such as oak, birch and juniper). The summer type is often induced by grass pollen (e.g., Bermuda, sweet vernal, orchard) and/or weed pollen (e.g., sheep sorrel, plantain). The fall type is generally a response to such weed pollens as ragweed and chamiso. Sometimes this type of hay fever is caused by airborne fungus spores.

b) Non-seasonal hay fever or allergic rhinitis may result from inhalation of irritants such as hay, straw, house dust and animal danders. It also can be caused by sensitivity to aspirin and other drugs. Possible sensitivity to foods and to food additives such as sodium benzoate, tartrazine yellow and MSG should be evaluated.

Note: Allergic rhinitis may lead to an increased susceptibility to other respiratory disorders, especially in polluted environments. Diarrhea, gas and indigestion are not uncommon in rhinitis, as the histamine response which is aggravating the sinus passages can also irritate the gastrointestinal tract.

BIOLOGICAL OVERVIEW

People with rhinitis notice that some years they are symptom-free and other years they suffer miserably. They also see a correlation between the severity of symptoms and their stress and health levels. Once these observations are made and corrective steps are taken, symptoms disappear. The hyper-reactivity of the sinuses and nasal membranes is directly related to overall health.

Sinus tissue reflects the health and structure of the head, teeth, nasal passages and jaw. Sometimes rhinitis indicates that a structural problem is impeding drainage. Cranio-sacral work can correct such obstructions. If polyps are present, surgical corrections may be necessary.

In most cases the sinuses are responding to local stress, whether from environmental pollens, air pollution (increasingly common), food sensitivity or irritation in related facial areas. Some cases of sinus inflammation can result from mercury sensitivity as minute amounts of mercury are released from dental amalgam fillings. Other sinus congestion can have its origin in a congested gut.

EMOTIONAL INFORMATION

Rhinitis frequently results from confusion. It sometimes arises in situations of unreleased anger, frustration or restriction of creative thoughts. Awareness and expression in words and action are important.

Hay fever often arises for the first time as an indicator of an "overload" situation: one pollen too many or one demand too many, as the case may be. In families with an extensive history of hay fever, habit can play a part. It can be difficult to withdraw from a seasonal family ritual of sneezing and pain.

GUIDELINES FOR ACTION

1. Avoid the allergens if possible.
2. Relieve inflammation of the sinuses, eyes, nose and throat.

3. Stimulate natural antihistamine responses in the nose and gut.
4. Enhance the liver's detoxifying action.
5. Support the adrenal glands.
6. Diagnose and eliminate chronic infection.
7. Eliminate abusive habits (the use of alcohol, drugs, caffeine, sugar; getting insufficient rest) which debilitate the immune system and the whole body.
8. Desensitize yourself prior to a hay fever season.

THERAPEUTICS RECOMMENDATIONS
FOODS

Chronic sinusitis often relates to food sensitivity and/or a low-grade infection. If your family history includes sinusitis, hay fever, arthritis, asthma, dermatitis, lupus SLE, depression and/or other psychiatric disorders, there is a good chance that dairy foods and/or grains may be irritating to your sinuses and other tissues. Eliminate these and substitute low-fat, high-fiber, vitamin-rich foods. Some examples: black or other beans, dark leafy greens, carrots, sweet potatoes, trout, salmon, bluefish, sardines, organic chicken and turkey and fresh fruits and vegetables. Cut back on sugar and sweets (the latter are usually high fat items as well). We have seen decades-long conditions of sinusitis clear with the elimination of wheat, in some cases. Sometimes goat products (goat cheese, milk, yogurt) will be tolerated when cow dairy is not. Goat's milk is more astringent and often less congestive than cow's milk.

In children, check for dark circles under the eyes, bright red ears, and a glassy look just as they go into a mood switch. These signs can indicate a food sensitivity. Frequently the elimination of heavily eaten favorite foods will help greatly. Other non-toxic favorites must be discovered, though, for the sanity of all concerned. Sometimes a Feingold diet is useful: preservative-free, additive free, low in salicylates. See Appendix F, p. 149 for more salicylate information.

If the sinus or hay fever condition is set off by a chronic infection, foods rich in vitamins A and C are essential (see Appendices). Also emphasize foods rich in protein and high zinc foods like sunflower seeds, pumpkin seeds and mushrooms. Shitake mushrooms are a specific for strengthening the immune system.

BASIS OF THERAPEUTICS

Foods with high fat content tend to clog the lymphatic system, increasing congestion, and should therefore be avoided. Low-fat, high-fiber foods promote a clearer lymphatic system and easier digestion.

Allergenic foods and chemicals can specifically irritate body tissues and cause malabsorption of needed nutrients. More information on this can be found in *Your Family Tree Connection* by Dr. Christopher Reed (see Bibliography).

Vitamins A and C and zinc stimulate the immune system. (See THE COMMON COLD, p. 22).

Shitake mushrooms (*Lentinus edodes*) contain antiviral compounds which increase interferon production.

BOTANICALS

Acute Formula

Ma Huang	6 parts	Take as an extract 20-40 drops every 2-3 hours during acute phase for symptomatic relief.
Eyebright	3 parts	
Yerba Santa	3 parts	
Yerba Mansa	3 parts	
Cayenne	1 part	

Balancing Formula

| Nettles (in | 6 parts | Take as a combined extract |
| fresh form | | 30 drops 3 times a day for 2- |

only)		4 months as a mucus mem-
Coltsfoot (in	4 parts	brane tonic. May be
fresh form		resumed when necessary.
only)		
Licorice	3 parts	
Toadflax	3 parts	
Barberry	2 parts	
Spikenard	2 parts	
Ginger	1 part	

Siberian Ginseng: 20 drops, 3 times a day for 2-4 months. May be resumed or continued if needed.

Fresh local bee pollen: Start taking the pollen at least 2 months before the hay fever season starts. Use just a tiny pinch at the start. If no reaction (e.g., constricted throat, teary eyes, shortness of breath, itchy skin), increase to 1 teaspoonful a day for a period of 2 weeks. If reactive, go back to using a tiny pinch until the reaction subsides, then very slowly increase to 1 teaspoon a day. This process may take up to 2-3 months. Take your time. (Pollen should be refrigerated.)

Warning: Always begin with a tiny pinch when starting a new batch of bee pollen, since it may contain a pollen to which you may be sensitive.

BASIS OF THERAPEUTICS

Ma Huang: Contains ephedrine which has adrenaline-like activity. Produces vasoconstriction of the mucous membranes, which reduces symptoms of congestion.

Eyebright: Decreases hyperactivity of the fixed antibodies found in the membranes of the throat, nose, eyes and ears. Specific for itchy, teary eyes and runny nose.

Yerba Santa: Helps dry out excess mucous production. Stimulates upper respiratory tissue repair.

Yerba Mansa: Contains caffeic acid glycosides which help strengthen the nasal tissues under stress.

Cayenne: Acts as a peripheral blood circulating stimulant. Helps moisten hot dry mucous membranes. Gives relief to frontal headaches caused by dry sinuses.

Nettles: Must be used in fresh or fresh freeze-dried forms; dried will not work. It is a specific for allergic rhinitis. Helps stabilize mast cells, thus breaking the vicious cycle of inflammation and hyperactivity of mucous membranes. A powerful antihistamine.

Coltsfoot: Must be used in fresh or fresh freeze-dried forms; dried will not work. Used with nettles, they are mutually reinforcing. Calms irritated mucous membranes. Also a potent antihistamine.

Licorice: Anti-inflammatory. Gives adrenal support. Acts as a synergist with other herbs.

Toadflax: A reliable liver stimulant. Helps the liver to break down inflammatory compounds such as histamine.

Barberry: Stimulates the liver's ability to de-activate inflammatory compounds and enhances its detoxification process.

Spikenard: Stops excessive mucous production.

Ginger: Acts as a tonic on the mucous membranes. A small amount adds energy to the other herbs.

Siberian Ginseng: An adrenal support. A very potent adaptogen for stressful situations.

Bee Pollen: Rich in B vitamins, especially pantothenic acid (see Supplements below). A good desensitizing agent.

SUPPLEMENTS

Vitamin C: 1,000-12,000 mg. per day after meals.

Pantothenic acid: 100 mg. per day, taken the month before and during hay fever season as a preventive.

Pantothenic acid: 250-500 mg. 3 times per day after meals during acute sinusitis or hay fever.

Calcium: 500 mg. per day at bedtime.

Magnesium: 500 mg. per day after a meal.

Bioflavonoids, especially Quercitin: 1,000-1,500 mg. per day to be taken with vitamin C.

A Good Multiple Vitamin and Mineral Formula: see Appendix D, p. 146.

Zinc (gluconate or chelated): 30-50 mg. once per day after a large meal.

Essential fatty acids, linseed, flaxseed or Max EPA™: 1,000-5,000 mg. (in capsules or oil) per day after meals.

BASIS OF THERAPEUTICS

Vitamin C: A potent antihistamine. Increases host resistance to secondary infection.

Pantothenic acid: A powerful antihistamine. Enhances immune function through macrophages and killer cells. Strengthens sinus and gut tissue.

Calcium: Calms inflammation.

Magnesium: Calms inflammation and relaxes nerves.

Bioflavinoids: Antihistamine. Some are antiviral, particularly Quercitin.

A Good Multiple Vitamin and Mineral Formula: Provides immune support with B-complex, beta-carotene and selenium.

Zinc: A strong immune system supporter. It enhances the activity of T-cells and T-helper cells in chronic and acute infection.

Essential fatty acids: Anti-inflammatory action.

PREVENTION AND HEALING

If this is your first bout with hay fever or sinusitis, this is the time to look carefully at your lifestyle. Alcohol and smoking greatly aggravate sinusitis, as do stress, overwork and a polluted environment.

A regimen of nettle extract, bioflavonoids (especially

quercitin) and pantothenic acid will take care of most mild cases of acute rhinitis.

If the condition is one of long standing, deeper balancing and a review of potential food sensitivities is in order. Acupuncture, exercise and a good diet with supportive herbs can make the difference between shortness of breath and sleeplessness and life with free breathing.

People who use topical decongestants may become dependent on them. Continued use produces, aggravates or perpetuates chronic rhinitis (also called rhinitis medicamentosa). Each time the decongestant is discontinued, a rebound congestion occurs. The best way to break this cycle is to stop "cold turkey." In several days you will breathe properly again. Get medical or health care support in this process if you feel you need it.

Clean air; clean air filter

Exercise.

VISUALIZATION

Acute hay fever: You are floating down a river on a raft. It is a warm soothing day. You breathe in fully and joyfully. What a pleasure it is to fully smell nature.

Chronic sinusitis or rhinitis: Think of all the people, conditions, issues you are angry about. Blow them out of the top of your head like a giant puff of smoke from a dragon— with power. Then see what is left in the sinus area—the hurt, the confusion, the joy. Soothe the area with whatever color or sound or touch feels most healing to you now.

NOTES

EARACHE (OTITIS MEDIA)

DEFINITION

Otitis media is a bacterial or viral infection of the middle ear. It usually follows an upper respiratory infection such as the flu, sinusitis, or sore throat.

DESCRIPTION

Otitis media is most common in young children, particularly from three months to three years of age. It usually starts with another infection such as a common cold and spreads to the middle ear via the eustachian tube mucous membrane. All respiratory infections can trigger otitis media and, therefore, should be promptly treated.

The first symptom usually is a persistent severe earache. Some hearing loss may occur. There can also be nausea, vomiting, diarrhea and fever (up to 105 degrees F. or 40.5 C.). Young children may tug or rub their ears to try to get some relief. Sometimes there will be a discharge from the ear. If not promptly and thoroughly treated, otitis media may result in serious complications, such as acute mastoiditis or recurrences of otitis media, and may require the first of many rounds of antibiotics.

BIOLOGICAL OVERVIEW

The air pressure in the middle ear is maintained at atmospheric levels by the eustachian tube. This tube opens into the nasal passages which connect with the mastoid bone (located behind the ear opening in the back part of the middle ear). This explains the ease with which a bacterium or virus may travel from the nose or sinus to the middle ear, causing an ear infection. This process is facilitated in young children because their eustachian tube is more horizontal than that of adults, permitting an even easier access. Once the middle ear is infected, the mastoid air cells are at risk because of their proximity. During the infection, inflammation can close the

Anatomy of the Ear

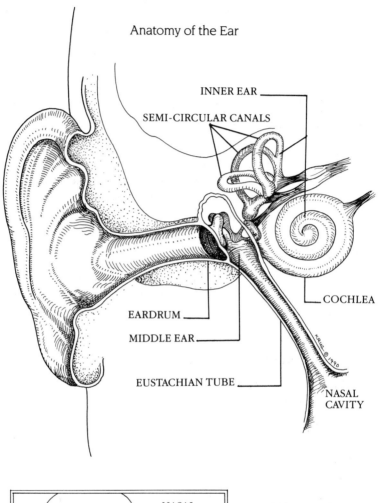

INNER EAR

SEMI-CIRCULAR CANALS

COCHLEA

EARDRUM

MIDDLE EAR

EUSTACHIAN TUBE

NASAL CAVITY

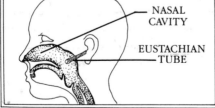

NASAL CAVITY

EUSTACHIAN TUBE

eustachian tube. Fluids may accumulate in the middle ear, causing nausea, vomiting and hearing loss. As a child grows, the eustachian tubes become more vertical. This anatomical change reduces the likelihood of ear infections and subsequent mastoiditis.

EMOTIONAL INFORMATION

There may be an unconscious desire to block out what is being said in the family, for example, parents fighting, angry words, or criticism. Parents need to consider that their child may be more aware than they realize. It is important to communicate love and reassurance to children. Sometimes underlying fear can be present in the child and the family.

GUIDELINES FOR ACTION

1. Treat all upper respiratory infections promptly.
2. Reduce inflammation of the eustachian tube and inner ear.
3. Increase drainage of accumulated fluids.
4. Strengthen the immune system.
5. If antibiotics are used, replenish the gastrointestinal microflora.
6. Prevent scarring of tissues.

THERAPEUTIC RECOMMENDATIONS
FOODS

Alkalizing (i.e., healing) foods include hot naturally sweetened lemonade (some flavorsome frozen lemonades are sweetened only with grape juice concentrate) and fresh carrot juice, orange juice, the latter two taken at room temperature; and the "Hot Brew for Colds" (see THE COMMON COLD/INFLUENZA, p. 21). Carrot sticks, squash, baked potatoes, spinach and pumpkin also are helpful.

If your breastfeeding child develops an earache,

eliminating dairy foods and sweets from your diet can help. In some children, earache is a symptom of food sensitivity. Eggs and dairy products are common offenders. If you want to minimize the infection, this is not the time to drink hot chocolate or give it to your child.

For more information see also COMMON COLD/INFLUENZA, p. 19.

BASIS OF THERAPEUTICS

Alkalizing foods, especially those rich in vitamins A and C such as those recommended above, support the immune system and speed healing. Warm foods are especially helpful for earache.

See also THE COMMON COLD/INFLUENZA, p. 19.

Why earaches may be a symptom of food sensitivity is not clearly understood, yet the connection frequently has been noted by pediatricians. Here is a possible explanation. Manganese, the essential trace mineral, provides support particularly for the inner and middle ear. When manganese is deficient, the inner ear is more likely to become inflamed. Manganese frequently is deficient in people with allergies. The reason for this is not yet known, but the connection is striking.

BOTANICALS

Licorice	6 parts	Take as a syrup ½ to 1
Mormon Tea	4 parts	teaspoon every 3-4 hours.
Yerba Santa	3 parts	
Eyebright	3 parts	
Echinacea	2 parts	
Ma Huang	1 part	
Cinnamon	1 part	

1 ounce Mullein Oil plus 6 drops of garlic oil, mix and refrigerate: drop 2-3 drops of warmed oil gently into each ear.

Licorice: A good anti-inflammatory. Makes a syrup palatable.

Mormon Tea: Contains small amounts of pseudoephedrine, making it a safe decongestant for children. Helps shrink swollen mucous membranes.

Yerba Santa: Decreases fluid production and shrinks inflamed tissues.

Eyebright: Inhibits inflammation of mucous membranes, especially of the eyes and middle ear.

Echinacea: Stimulates the immune system. Increases fluid resorption in the middle ear.

Ma Huang: A decongestant.

Cinnamon: Helps reduce symptoms of nausea, vomiting and diarrhea. Also makes the syrup more flavorful.

Mullein & Garlic Oil: Balances pH of ear, prevents infection, warms and soothes the ear tissue.

SUPPLEMENTS

FOR ADULTS: Same as Common Cold with the addition of:

Manganese gluconate or chelate: 50 mg. once per day after a meal.

Vitamin E: 400-800 I.U. per day after a meal.

Linseed oil capsules (essential fatty acids): 1250-2500 mg. per day after meals.

FOR CHILDREN: Beta-carotene: 5,000 I.U. once per day. (Lemon grass beta-carotene is available in this lower potency.)

Zinc lozenges: 15-23 mg. twice a day after meals.

Chewable buffered vitamin C: 250 mg. every hour, 3,000 mg. per day maximimum.

A Good Multiple Vitamin and Mineral Formula: see page 146.

Liquid garlic (odorless): 15 drops 3 times per day in juice.

Manganese gluconate: 5-25 mg. per day after a meal.

Chewable vitamin E: 100-200 I.U. per day.

Linseed oil capsules or liquid (essential fatty acids): 1,000 mg. once or twice per day after a meal.

BASIS OF THERAPEUTICS

Manganese: Essential for support of the inner and middle ear. Calms inflammation and speeds healing.

Linseed Oil (essential fatty acids): Works with manganese to calm inflammation in the middle ear. A flaky, crusty buildup in the outer ear is a specific indication of essential fatty acid deficiency.

Vitamin E: Is most appropriately used in cases of recurrent otitis media. It helps prevent the scarring of tissues in the eustachian tubes, which can lead to loss of hearing.

See THE COMMON COLD/INFLUENZA (p. 22) for explanation of the remaining supplements.

PREVENTION AND HEALING

If your child has had repeated earaches, you should consider having her/him checked for food allergies by a competent specialist. An excess intake of sugar also can cause recurrent otitis media.

As we explained in the Biological Overview, usually children will outgrow episodes of otitis media as their eustachian tubes become more vertical. Some pediatricians have found that acupuncture helps children to heal faster and prevents recurrences of the infection. A supportive family environment, attention to possible food sensitivities, and long-term prevention of infection (see COMMON COLD/INFLUENZA, p. 23) are effective healing measures. Make sure head, feet and back are protected and kept warm at all times.

It has been observed that children who have taken antibiotics once are more susceptible to recurrences of middle ear infection. Therefore, it is extremely important to re-establish proper gastrointestinal microflora after a course of antibiotics. Life Start (manufactured by Natren) is a bifido bacterium (a type of acidophilus) which speeds up microflora replacement and strengthens the immune system. Licorice tea, which prevents candidiasis, may be given for three to four months following the infection. It also supports the adrenal glands in the secretion of anti-inflammatory compounds.

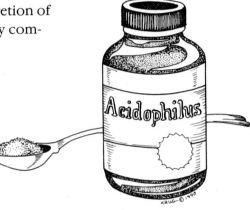

HEALING PROCESS

Rub your hands briskly together until they are quite warm. Take in a deep breath, then place one hand over each ear. Breath out gently. Breath in and out five or six times, leaving your hands on your ears. Experience the feelings of warmth and security as you do this.

SORE THROATS

DEFINITION

Sore throat is an inflammation of the pharynx, larynx and/or upper trachea.

DESCRIPTION

Sore throats may be of an acute or a chronic nature.

a)   Acute sore throat usually is caused by bacterial or viral infection. It can occur alone or in association with pharyngitis, acute rhinitis or other upper respiratory infections. It also may occur with the flu, pneumonia, bronchitis, measles, diphtheria, or as a result of inhalation of irritants. The main symptoms are hoarseness, pain, rawness or a tickling sensation in the throat, malaise, and in some cases, fever. A cough also may be present.

b)   Chronic sore throat may be caused by repeated acute inflammations, chronic abuse of the vocal cords, repeated or sustained inhalation of irritants (including smoking), chronic sinus or throat infections, or allergies. In rare instances laryngitis may be an indication of syphilis or tuberculosis. The main symptoms of chronic sore throats are hoarseness, cough, expectoration of thick mucus and a feeling of dryness in the throat.

BIOLOGICAL OVERVIEW

A sore throat or a low grade fever may be the first sign that your body is in need of rest, that it is fighting for your well being, or that it is overloaded with toxins. If this condition is not given immediate attention it may progress to a strep throat or a full-blown cold, for which antibiotics may be needed. By taking care of yourself and resting, you free all of the body's available energy to fight the approaching disease.

Sweating is one of the surest ways to lower a fever and to eliminate waste products.

EMOTIONAL INFORMATION

Sore throats often occur when we are angry at ourselves or others and have not expressed this anger. Laryngitis frequently manifests as we are backing away from something—an important creative opportunity, overwork, or a difficult situation in which we have been reluctant to speak out. Laryngitis can provide a useful retreat to regroup our forces or an avoidance/escape. The loss of voice in laryngitis also can be an extension of the anger of a sore throat or express a need for a period of silence.

GUIDELINES FOR ACTION

1. Rest

2. Decrease inflammation of the throat.

3. Stimulate the immune system.

4. Eliminate any infection.

5. Avoid irritants, especially if the condition is chronic: tobacco smoke, alcohol, dust, fumes, allergens and air pollutants.

6. Humidify and soothe the tissues.

THERAPEUTIC RECOMMENDATIONS
FOODS

First and foremost use alkalizing foods as described in THE COMMON COLD/ INFLUENZA p. 19.

Small amounts of astringent and pungent foods also can be useful. An effective example of this is the following healing tea:* 1 clove of raw garlic pressed, juice of 1 fresh lemon, a pinch or $\frac{1}{16}$ tsp. cayenne, 1 tsp. honey, combined in 1 cup boiled water. Sip as often as you can handle it.

Astringent foods (and juices made from them) such as fresh oranges, lemons, limes, grapefruits, kiwis and pomegranates are recommended as a supplement to fruits advised in THE COMMON COLD/INFLUENZA, p. 19.

*This formulation contributed by Shamaan Ochaum, a health-care practitioner in Austin, Texas.

Increase fluids, using up to 2-3 qts. per day, warm or hot. These may be sweetened with honey or maple syrup.

BASIS OF THERAPEUTICS

Alkalizing foods discourage viral spread. Mildly astringent foods, especially in combination with the herbs recommended above, help to reduce the engorgement of the mucosa characteristic of sore throats. Those listed also are rich in natural ascorbic acid (vitamin C).

Fluids are increased because they soothe and humidify throat tissue, thereby speeding healing.

Honey relieves congestion, soothes the throat and provides a mild astringency to reduce engorged tissues. Maple syrup is more specifically cooling and is recommended for individuals who tend to be "fiery" (i.e., those with hot tempers and a history of skin rashes, stomach ulcers, or other inflammations). Cayenne increases circulation to stressed tissues. Garlic provides immune support and slows the growth of viruses. The latter two supports should be used very moderately by excessively fiery types.

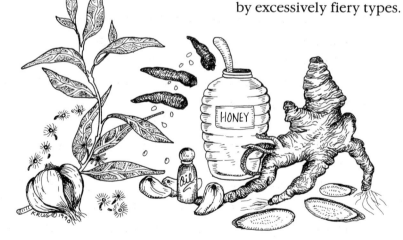

BOTANICALS

| Collinsonia | 6 parts | See next page for rest of |
| Stillingia | 5 parts | formula |

Propolis	4 parts	Take as a combined extract
Echinacea	4 parts	20-40 drops in sufficient
Osha	3 parts	water to gargle. Swallow
Licorice	2 parts	after gargling. Repeat every
Marshmallow	2 parts	3 hours.
Yerba Mansa	2 parts	
Poke Root	1 part	
Blood Root	1 part	

BASIS OF THERAPEUTICS

Collinsonia: Specific herb for sore throats and laryngitis. Stimulates blood circulation in the throat. Specifically prevents middle ear inflammation.

Stillingia: Increases lymph drainage from subcutaneous and sub-mucosal tissues. Stimulates hydration of the throat.

Propolis: Prevents bacterial invasion of the throat. Slows down replication of viruses. Decreases inflammation of the larynx.

Echinacea: Stimulates immune system response.

Osha: Decreases inflammation of the respiratory tissues. Stimulates production and excretion of thin mucus.

Licorice: Decreases inflammation and soothes irritated tissues. Synergistic to other herbs.

Marshmallow: Soothes inflamed throat tissue.

Yerba Mansa: Adds strength to the tissues, thus preventing ulceration.

Poke Root: Decreases inflammation of the lymph nodes. Acts with Echinacea to stimulate immune response.

Blood Root: Increases blood flow through injured tissues. *Warning:* Should be used in very small amounts. Can be toxic.

SUPPLEMENTS

Beta-carotene—30,000-100,000 I.U. per day total, taken after meals for no more than 5 days. See the warning note in ABOUT SUPPLEMENTS, p. 8.

Zinc lozenges—15 mg. 5 times per day for the first 5 days; 3 times per day thereafter.

BASIS FOR THERAPEUTICS

Zinc: Is specific for sore throats. It provides topical anti-viral action. Chronic throat infections often indicate a zinc deficiency. Thirty to forty milligrams of zinc daily after meals for 2-3 months can remedy this. Zinc deficiency is more common among people on low protein, vegetarian and/or high bran diets.

A Good Multiple Vitamin and Mineral Formula: Addresses possible thyroid imbalances caused by shortages of iodine, copper, zinc, magnesium and tyrosine. A chronic sore throat can indicate a thyroid disorder: check with a trusted health care practitioner.

Beta-carotene: In addition to its immune enhancing actions, provides support for the throat chronically abused by excess alcohol and/or tobacco.

See also THE COMMON COLD/INFLUENZA, p. 22.

PREVENTION AND HEALING

At the first signs of sore throat, gargle hourly with echinacea and osha (20 drops each of the tincture in ½ glass warm water, to be swallowed after). Salt water gargles (1 Tbsp. sea salt per 4 oz. warm water) on rising and at bedtime also are recommended. Gargle, do not swallow. These in addition to zinc lozenges slowly dissolved in the throat up to 5 times a day will often effectively head off a sore throat.

Express your feelings freely. Rest. A eucalyptus oil steam inhalation is very soothing and speeds recovery. A non-narcotic cough syrup may be used to relieve nonproductive coughs.

Soothing foods rich in vitamin A—carrot juice, dark leafy greens, sweet potatoes—can calm the throat and speed healing.

Chewing on licorice and/or osha root is soothing to sore throats.

If the condition has become chronic, it is extremely important to examine your over-all lifestyle. Do you smoke? Do you drink alcohol daily? Do you frequent smoke-filled environments? Are you over-using your voice? These abuses must be addressed.

Are you involved in frustrating situations you have hesitated to speak out about? Perhaps you have avoided admitting your frustration even to yourself. These repressed feelings need to be examined.

Rest, exercise in fresh air and self-nurturing are essential.

VISUALIZATION

You are standing at the base of a large and beautiful waterfall. As you breathe in the cool soothing spray, you can hear the sounds of the water as it dances against the rocks. Imagine how the rocks feel as the water gently flows down and around them.

COUGHS

DEFINITION

A cough is a sudden and forceful expiration of air from the lungs.

DESCRIPTION

Coughing can be symptomatic of various disorders. Therefore, the cause of a cough must be identified and specifically treated. Coughs may accompany asthma, acute and chronic bronchitis, allergies, diphtheria, uterus irritation, middle ear inflammation, pharyngitis, laryngitis and influenza. Diaphragm, stomach or intestinal irritation, whooping cough (pertussis), congestive heart failure and mitral valve disease also can produce a cough.

BIOLOGICAL OVERVIEW

Coughing is normally a protective phenomenon. It is the most common symptom of a respiratory disease. Any irritation occurring in the area between the upper throat and the terminal bronchioles may initiate a cough. It usually serves to expel excretions or foreign materials from the respiratory tract. When it is productive (i.e., when mucus comes up), it should not be suppressed. It should be stopped only if it is exhausting the person or when it is absolutely non-productive. A dry cough needs moisture, which can be provided with steam and fluids; a wet cough needs dryness, such as a dry sauna, pungent foods and herbs.

Because coughs stem from a variety of causes, there is no single course of therapy. Treating the causative disease appropriately usually will resolve the cough.

EMOTIONAL INFORMATION

Coughs generally indicate that there is something you need to "get off your chest," often something irritating, painful or constricting. Relief may come simply from expressing your feelings about it.

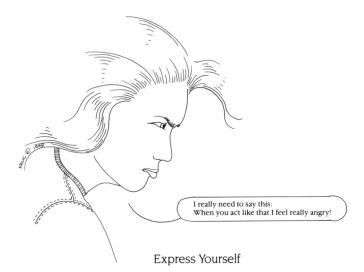

I really need to say this:
When you act like that I feel really angry!

Express Yourself

GUIDELINES FOR ACTION

1. Secure proper diagnosis.

2. Support the throat, lungs and any other irritated tissues.

3. Stimulate the immune system.

4. Rest.

5. Decrease irritation to the brain nerve-cough center (medulla oblongata).

6. Increase fluids and electrolytes (see p. 132) if vomiting accompanies cough.

THERAPEUTIC RECOMMENDATIONS

The causes that precipitate the cough must be identified and dealt with thoroughly.

The following suggestions are primarily symptomatic therapies.

FOODS

Coughs generally indicate congestion in the lungs. East Indian medicine (Ayurveda) suggests that certain foods, especially sweets, increase congestion in the lungs and, when taken over a long period, promote coughs. Dairy foods (especially ice cream), and in some cases wheat, also can contribute to this congestion. It is recommended to avoid sweets and choose foods rich in vitamins A and C (see Appendix C, p. 133).

See also Foods, THE COMMON COLD, p. 19 and ACUTE BRONCHITIS, p. 69.

Increase fluids up to 2-3 quarts per day if the cough is dry. If it is wet, maintain at 1-2 quarts per day of mainly clear broths and teas which may be sweetened with honey.

Pungent foods, such as onion, garlic, leeks, ginger, chili peppers and Indian curries are helpful in breaking up the congestion.

BASIS OF THERAPEUTICS

From a Western perspective, sweets acidify the system, promote viral growth and congest the lymphatics. From an Ayurvedic perspective, sweets and dairy foods (as they are served in this country, cold and pasteurized) promote the build-up of excess heaviness and moisture in the lungs. Avoiding them helps to prevent this condition.

Pungent foods and spices enhance circulation to the lungs as well as to the body as a whole. They warm a cold system, break up congestion, promote expectoration and get fluids moving.

BOTANICALS

Osha	4 parts	Take as a syrup ½ to 1
Wild Cherry bark	3 parts	teaspoon every 3-4 hours
White Pine bark	3 parts	as needed.
Licorice	2 parts	
Balm of Gilead	1 part	
Spikenard	1 part	
Blood Root	1 part	

Passion flower: 20-40 drops of extract every 2-3 hours as needed.

BASIS OF THERAPEUTICS

Osha: Reduces inflammation of the mucous membranes. It also quickly soothes and anesthetizes these tissues.

Wild Cherry bark: Contains prunasin, which acts as a mild sedative to the irritated mucous membranes of the throat.

White Pine bark: A useful expectorant. It modifies favorably the quality and quantity of the mucus secretions.

Licorice: A good anti-inflammatory. Mediates effectiveness of the other herbs in a formula.

Balm of Gilead: Acts as an anti-inflammatory. Contains low amounts of salicin, a precursor of aspirin.

Spikenard: Stimulates phagocytosis in white blood cells. Some herbalists hypothesize that Spikenard stimulates infected cells to increase their synthesis of interferon.

Bloodroot: In small doses it activates blood circulation, especially at the site of stagnation. Speeds up healing of the injured tissues.

Passion flower: A specific for coughs caused by excessive irritation of the cough center in the brain stem. (The cough irritates the brain stem which in turn intensifies the cough: a commonly occurring vicious circle.)

SUPPLEMENTS

Beta-carotene: If acute: 30,000-100,000 I.U./day (TOTAL) for up to 5 days. No more than 15,000 total I.U. if you are pregnant or trying to conceive. See ABOUT SUPPLEMENTS, p. 9.

If chronic: 10,000-30,000 I.U. per day.

Vitamin E: 400 I.U. 1-2 times per day after meals.

Buffered vitamin C: 1,000-10,000 mg. per day.

A Good Multiple Vitamin and Mineral Formula: Choose

one that is rich in B vitamins, especially if dealing with whooping cough.

Zinc lozenges: 15 mg. 5 times per day for the first 5 days and 2-3 times per day thereafter. For children, 15 mg. 3 times a day maximum.

Garlic: 1 capsule 3-5 times per day with meals.

Caprylic acid: If the causative condition is yeast related, see FUNGAL RESPIRATORY INFECTIONS p. 102.

BASIS OF THERPEUTICS

Beta-carotene: Supports the immune system and acts as a preventive, discouraging potential infections from developing

Vitamin E: Enhances flexibility and moisture of the lung membranes. 800 I.U. per day can help calm inflammation; 400 I.U. per day generally will not.

Buffered vitamin C: Supports the immune system.

A Good Multiple Vitamin and Mineral Formula well supplied with B complex and especially including folic acid is useful in discouraging bacterial infections. May be especially helpful in dealing with whooping cough, an infection caused by a particularly virulent gram-negative bacteria unresponsive to antibiotics.

Zinc: Promotes localized immune defense through mobilization of T-cells and lymphocytes.

Garlic: Warms and breaks up congestion. Promotes immune function.

PREVENTION AND HEALING

Notice when and where your cough occurs. This can lead to the discovery and avoidance of allergenic foods and substances which precipitated the cough. Do you begin to cough after you eat corn? Does your child cough more when you put him/her down for a nap? She/he may be reacting to a filler in the bedding or in the stuffed toys there. Animal danders also can promote a coughing attack. Additional support includes:

1. Bed rest.

2. Humidifier if dry cough.

3. Dry sauna if wet cough.

VISUALIZATION

You are in a quiet soothing space. You have all the support you need around you. You take a deep breath and fill your lungs completely. The air soothes each cell. You let it out, expelling the built-up wastes. Repeat this as often and as slowly as you need.

PLEURISY

DEFINITION

Pleurisy is an inflammation of the lubricating lining that covers the lungs. The diaphragm and the walls of the chest cavity also are lined with lubricating tissue which can become inflamed.

DESCRIPTION

The symptoms of pleurisy are chilliness, fever, stabbing pain or stitch on the affected side, sharp pain when coughing or breathing deeply. The fever ranges between 101° and 103°F. (38.3° to 39.4°C.). There often is pain between the ribs, under the lower margin of the ribs and into the abdomen. There also can be pain from the shoulders to the neck and along the sternum. Usually relief is experienced when the person lies on the affected side. Pleurisy often follows another respiratory infection, such as the common cold or pneumonia. This demonstrates the importance of attending to all infection immediately.

BIOLOGICAL OVERVIEW

The role of the pleura is to reduce friction between the outer layers of the lungs and the chest cavity during breathing. In pleurisy these linings become inflamed and congested and stop lubricating the tissues. When the person breathes, this lack of lubrication produces a sharp stabbing pain. She/he tends to breath shallowly and rapidly to avoid coughing. Another way to minimize the pain is to hold the ribs to restrict movement.

If the inflammatory process continues, an accumulation of fluids can build up in the chest cavity. It is important that waste products from the lungs be properly eliminated. Therefore cough-suppressing drugs or herbs should not be given, as these may contribute to a secondary bacterial infection (see COUGH, p. 47).

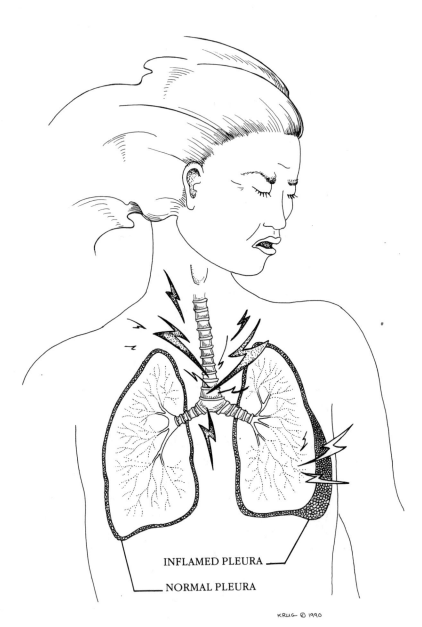

INFLAMED PLEURA

NORMAL PLEURA

KRUG © 1990

Pain Caused by Pleurisy

EMOTIONAL INFORMATION

Subtle and unnoticed patterns of self-neglect can underlie this condition. There may be a tendency to over-extend emotionally and physically. Situations may be "rubbing you the wrong way." Allowing the time and space to meet your own needs is important.

GUIDELINES FOR ACTION

1. Reduce inflammation of the pleura.
2. Assure proper hydration.
3. Increase lymphatic drainage of the pleural cavity.
4. Maintain electrolyte levels.
5. Support production of quality lubricants by pleural membranes.
6. Support and normalize respiration.

THERAPEUTICS RECOMMENDATIONS
FOODS

Lots of warm fluids should be taken. Two to four cups of clear soup, healing broth (see p. 132) or the proverbial chicken noodle soup is vitally important to the healing process. Miso soup with onions, garlic and parsley is excellent. Shitake mushrooms may be added. Bernard Jensen's mineral broth (1 teaspoon per cup of hot water) and fresh vegetable juices also are helpful.

As is recommended for most respiratory illnesses, during the acute infectious stage the intake of dairy products should be reduced or stopped.

BASIS OF THERAPEUTICS

Fluids rehydrate the lungs. Onion, garlic, parsley and shitake mushrooms stimulate immune response. The healing broth (see p. 132) and Bernard Jensen's mineral broth replace electrolytes and lost fluids.

BOTANICALS

Hyssop oil: 2 drops in honey 3 times a day. The undiluted oil also can be used in a vaporizer/humidifier that has a well. Or add 5 drops of the oil to a bowl of hot water and inhale the steam keeping a towel over the head and bowl to hold in vapors.

Pleurisy root	6 parts	Take as a combined extract
Coltsfoot	5 parts	30-60 drops every 2 hours
Licorice	5 parts	during acute phase. Take
Mullein	4 parts	20 drops 3 times a day for 1
Osha	4 parts	month after disappearance
Echinacea	2 parts	of symptoms.
Inmortal	2 parts	
Virginia snakeroot	1 part	

BASIS OF THERAPEUTICS

Hyssop oil: Prevents stagnation of bronchial secretions.

Pleurisy Root: Increases fluid circulation and lymph drainage of inflamed tissues. Relieves blood congestion by stimulating the vagus nerve. Promotes quality secretion of serous fluids. Increases over-all humidity of the lungs.

Coltsfoot: An anti-inflammatory. Stabilizes mast cells, which are secretors of inflammatory compounds. Increases lymphatic drainage.

Licorice: Synergistic effects with other herbs. Also has an anti-inflammatory action.

Mullein: mild Anti-inflammatory.

Osha: Stimulates sweating, which increases elimination of toxins and reduces fevers. It helps pleural membranes utilize fluids more effectively.

Echinacea: Stimulates lymphatic drainage. Stimulates monocytes, thereby preventing infection. Stimulates macrophages which clear up debris.

Inmortal: Same actions as pleurisy root. Also has a

cardiac glycoside that strengthens and supports the heart.

Virginia Snakeroot: Stimulates blood flow in congested pulmonary tissues.

SUPPLEMENTS

Beta-carotene: 10,000-30,000 I.U. a day for no more than 5 days. See warning p. 9.

Vitamin C: 1,000-6,000 mg. a day, up to 500 mg. every hour.

Vitamin E: 400-800 I.U. once a day after a meal.

Zinc gluconate: 25 mg. 3 times a day after meals (maximum of 75 mg. elemental zinc).

A Good Multiple Vitamin and Mineral Formula or B-complex formula: as generally recommended for support (see p. 146).

Essential fatty acids: linseed, flax seeds or Max EPA™ 1,000 mg. capsules to be taken every 2 hours.

BASIS OF THERAPEUTICS

Beta-carotene: Stimulates lubrication of the pleural membranes. Replaces diseased membrane cells with healthy ones. Strengthens white blood cell immune action.

Vitamin C: As an antioxidant, supports membranes and connective tissues. Maintains oxygen turnover in respiration.

Vitamin E: Strengthens and lubricates membranes.

Zinc gluconate: Fights underlying infection through stimulation of T-cells and T-helper cells.

Essential fatty acids: Reduce inflammation by stimulating production of calming prostaglandin.

PREVENTION AND HEALING

1. Bed rest.

2. Humidifier: use 24 hours a day.

3. Keep well-hydrated.

4. The painful area can be bound with a cloth to limit aggravating movements. Lying on the side which hurts also alleviates pain. Binding is useful in most cases but should not be used by people with known prior pulmonary insufficiency (i.e., C.O.P.D.). In such cases binding could increase congestion of the lungs and thereby promote infection.

5. A poultice may be helpful. Grind flax seeds into a meal and mix with enough water to make a paste. Apply along the painful area of the rib cage, about ⅛" to ¼" thick. Clay also may be used. The poultice can be held in place with the binding cloth.

Pleurisy is often a one-time illness. It calls attention for the need to strengthen the body and also to take care of emotional needs. Do not neglect yourself. If there are recurrences, underlying nutritional deficiencies and/or chemical sensitivity or toxicity may be present. A thorough medical examination is recommended in such cases.

VISUALIZATION

Imagine a beautiful pink flower with thin transparent petals. As you breath in and out, imagine the petals of this flower getting thicker and thicker. They become a cool resilient cushion with fluids and air streaming in and out of them. Send this same love and nourishment to yourself.

PNEUMONIA

DEFINITION

Pneumonia is an inflammation of the alveolar spaces of the lungs. It usually occurs in response to bacterial, viral or chemical irritation. Debilitated or hospitalized patients can contract pneumonia as a result of a fungal or parasitic infection. *Pneumonia is a life-threatening disease and requires the skilled assistance of a physician.*

DESCRIPTION

More than 50 causative agents have been identified in pneumonia, the vast majority of which are of viral or bacterial origin. It is estimated that viral pneumonia accounts for a high percentage of all acute pulmonary infections. Children are at higher risk.

The symptoms of bacterial pneumonia are chills, high fever, chest pain, cough, sore throat, extreme weakness, muscle ache and, in some instances, blood in the sputum. Rapid and labored breathing, nausea, vomiting, fast pulse and malaise also may be present. In the aged and very young, the infection may not be accompanied by a fever. If oral herpes has been present, it may be reactivated.

Bacterial pneumonia is especially life-threatening. The onset of symptoms, which can be intense, usually is sudden. Medical attention should be sought immediately.

Viral pneumonia may produce no symptoms in some cases. In others there will be progressive breathing problems, fever, headache, muscle ache, and extreme tiredness. It can be mildly to highly contagious. Sputum is thicker and coughing and chest pains are less marked than in bacterial infections.

In both cases, there may be shallow, rapid breathing to compensate for low oxygen levels.

BIOLOGICAL OVERVIEW

Predisposing factors are contraction of the common

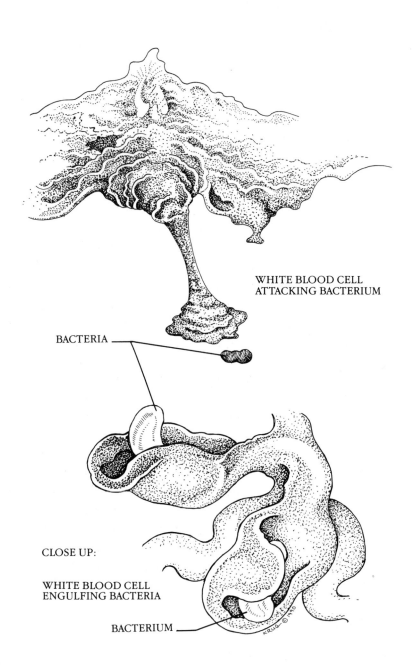

WHITE BLOOD CELL
ATTACKING BACTERIUM

BACTERIA

CLOSE UP:

WHITE BLOOD CELL
ENGULFING BACTERIA

BACTERIUM

cold or an upper respiratory infection, acute and chronic alcoholism, malnutrition, debility, exposure, treatment with immunosuppressive drugs and/or radiation. The aged, persons with chronic respiratory disease or heart failure, and post-operative patients are at risk. Poor blood circulation is a factor in bed-ridden people. Pneumonia is more prevalent in the winter months and in areas with polluted air.

Apparently pneumonia begins with bacteria or viruses entering into the lungs. In reality, the lungs, immune system, and/or adrenal glands probably have been gradually wearing down prior to the infection. Your body can use this opportunity to reverse these predisposing conditions and get healthy again.

Once the microorganisms have entered the lungs, the alveoli respond by producing an inflammatory exudate which isolates the intruders. This also signals the immune system to move into action. White blood cells then enter the area to defend the lungs and to engulf and break down the microorganisms. Finally, the body rids itself of the infectious debris and waste products through the lymphatic and blood systems. Now is the time for deeper healing.

EMOTIONAL INFORMATION

Often, you have been pushing too hard for too long. You may feel that certain conditions have been weighing down on you, of loss, grief or simple overwork. There is a strong need to create more space in your life—for you. You could consider this illness as a healing oasis, an opportunity to begin to put your life's priorities in a more realistic perspective. It is time to stop and rest and re-balance.

GUIDELINES FOR ACTION

1. Support the respiratory system (i.e., increase oxygen uptake).

2. Stimulate the immune system.

3. Reduce inflammation and increase drainage of the alveoli.

4. Increase blood flow through the lung tissues.

5. Normalize production of mucus.

6. Stimulate the cleansing system.

7. Support overall healing energy, especially of the adrenals.

THERAPEUTIC RECOMMENDATIONS

The following botanical and dietary suggestions in combination with orthodox treatment will hasten the healing and resolution of this condition.

FOODS

Foods rich in vitamins A, C and E are especially useful here. A healing broth (p. 132) prepared with broccoli, carrots, parsley, watercress, nettles, and/or other dark leafy greens will be supportive and strengthening. It can be taken two to three times per day.

At least 4 to 6 glasses of water and other fluids should be taken daily. Foods prepared with raw garlic also are helpful.

BASIS OF THERAPEUTICS

Healing Broth replenishes potassium and other electrolytes lost in the alveoli exudate.

Garlic prevents proliferation of pathogenic microorganisms.

Water and broth replenish lost fluids.

BOTANICALS

Chlorophyll concentrate: 20 drops, 3 times a day with meals.

Osha	4 parts
Eucalyptus leaves	4 parts
Inmortal	3 parts
Licorice	3 parts
Echinacea	2 parts
Grindelia	2 parts
Blood root	1 part

Take as a combined tincture. 40 to 60 drops every 2 hours in warm water.

BASIS OF THERAPEUTICS

Chlorophyll: Increases uptake of oxygen by the lungs and oxygenation of all body tissues.

Osha: Is one of the best herbal anti-viral agents. Helps reduce inflammation of the alveoli. Strengthens and stimulates cilia action in the bronchioles, thus helping clear mucus.

Eucalyptus: Its oils are exhaled through the lung tissues, thus inhibiting bacterial growth. It liquifies mucus and facilitates its expectoration.

Inmortal Root: Stimulates lymph flow in the alveolar tissues. It supports the right side of the heart (the side that pumps blood in the lungs). It also acts as a bronchial dilator.

Licorice: An excellent anti-inflammatory. Supports adrenal functions. The emulsifying properties of its saponins increase the absorption of other herbs.

Echinacea: Stimulates immune response by increasing chemotaxis of the white blood cells, thereby helping them get to the area of stress faster. Stimulates macrophages to cleanse the site of infection.

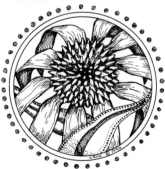

ECHINACEA FLOWER

Grindelia: Stimulates mucus expectoration and promotes alveolar repair.

Blood root: Increases blood flow in and out of the alveolar capillaries, thus enabling more nutrients to get to the needy cells of the injured area.

SUPPLEMENTS

Garlic: 1 or 2 pearls 3 times a day with meals.

Vitamin A (beta-carotene): 10,000-30,000 I.U. after meals 1 to 3 times a day for no more than 5 days.
See warning p. 9.

Vitamin C: 1,000-6,000 mg. daily as buffered ascorbate (500 mg. hourly). See warning p. 8.

Zinc: Lozenges to be dissolved in the mouth after meals. 25 mg. 3 times a day for the first 5 days, twice a day thereafter. Should not be taken on an empty stomach.

After resolution of the infection:
Vitamin E: 400 I.U. once a day after a meal.

Selenium: 200 mcg. once a day after a meal.

A Good Multiple Vitamin and Mineral Formula: see p. 146.

BASIS OF THERAPEUTICS

Garlic: see foods, p. 62.

Vitamin A: Supports white blood cell activity and rebuilds the mucosal lining of the lungs. Creates adrenal support during fatigue. Increases the strength of epithelial cells. Promotes tissue lubrication.

Vitamin C: Is particularly useful for viral pneumonia. Strengthens white blood cells. Stimulates the production of interferon, a natural anti-viral compound.

Zinc: Blocks replication of viruses. Regulates release of Vitamin A from the liver and stimulates its activity in the cells of the infected area.

Vitamin E: Acts as an antioxidant, strengthening the

white blood cells and tissue lining of the lung. It promotes the breakdown of toxic waste products and assists vitamin A metabolism.

Selenium: Useful in rebuilding lung tissue. Promotes liver action to break down toxic chemicals.

The Multiple Vitamin and Mineral Formula: Rebuilds an overall depleted system.

PREVENTION AND HEALING

Bed rest: It is essential that complete bed rest be maintained during the acute phase. Wait another 1 to 2 days after the fever subsides before getting out of bed. This will shorten the duration of the disease and prevent further complications.

Deep breathing: At least 3 or 4 deep breaths should be taken every hour. This will help insure adequate ventilation of the lungs, stimulates lymph drainage and accelerate healing.

Steam vaporizers: Use in preference to cool mist humidifiers. They prevent contamination from bacterial overgrowth and do not lower room temperature. Furthermore, they usually have a well which may be filled with healing oils such as eucalyptus or thyme.

This disease acts as a signal that healing and strengthening is needed throughout the body. Prompt attention to colds and flus is important. Rest and regular use of the nutrients and foods listed above and in THE COMMON COLD/INFLUENZA section, p. 19, are essential.

VISUALIZATION

Lie down in a quiet peaceful place. You can feel your head and body resting on a soft pink resilient cushion. It moves up and down with your breath. As you allow yourself to relax more deeply into these sensations of softness and receiving, you can feel a letting go happening in your whole body. As you let go, the feelings move up and out. Give yourself permission to relax and sleep. Rest in this place of light and strength.

NOTES

ACUTE BRONCHITIS

DEFINITION

Acute Bronchitis is an inflammation of the trachea and bronchi caused either by infection or irritation. It is generally self-limiting, and complete healing with a full return of function usually follows.

DESCRIPTION

There are two types of Acute Bronchitis.

a) Infectious: It occurs more frequently in winter. It may develop following a common cold or other upper respiratory infection. Recurrent attacks may suggest a focus of infection elsewhere in the body, such as in the sinuses, colon, or, in children, in the tonsils or adenoids. Repeated occurrences may also indicate allergies.

b) Irritative: It can be caused by inhalation of mineral or vegetable dust fumes, tobacco smoke, or other irritants.

Symptoms for both include malaise, chills, cough, back and muscle pain, sore throat and a fever of 100° to 102°F (37.8° to 38.9°C).

BIOLOGICAL OVERVIEW

Bronchitis is usually mild and resolves itself spontaneously. Smokers are at higher risk. If you are run-down, very young or have chronic pulmonary or cardiac disease, extra care is essential, as pneumonia is a potentially serious complication.

At first, the mucous membranes of the trachea and bronchi become congested. This impaired function may cause bacteria to invade the normally sterile bronchi. The lungs' protective reaction is: (1) to shed surface lining cells, (2) to induce inflammation, (3) to produce a protective mucus and (4) to send for white blood cells to counter the invasion.

The cough at first is dry and painful and later becomes productive with mucus and pus. As the inflammation subsides, cough and expectoration diminish and disappear. During the feverish and inflamed stage, water may be exhaled through the lungs at a rate of 3 to 4 quarts a day. Adequate intake of mineral-rich fluids is essential to replace this loss.

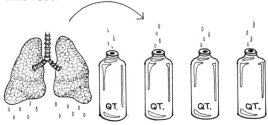

Water Loss by Lungs during Acute Inflammation

A rule of thumb in treating coughs: *if the cough is productive, do not suppress it.* An exception to this would be if the coughing has exhausted you and prevented sleep. If the cough is dry and nonproductive, cough suppressants may be considered. (See COUGHS for suggestions, p. 47.)

Strong cough suppressants, such as codeine, will inhibit mucus excretion and can prolong inflammation and infection of the lung tissues. Therefore, they should not be used.

Bronchial wall swelling, bronchial muscle spasms and mucus accumulation can cause airway obstructions. These conditions require prompt medical attention.

EMOTIONAL INFORMATION

A buildup of old feelings and ideas or outworn roles can contribute to acute bronchitis. The need to get something off your chest and/or a fear of opening to the new life and feelings before you also can be contributing factors. Bronchitis may be a signal that a release of old patterns and an opening to new ones should be initiated.

GUIDELINES FOR ACTION

1. Stimulate the pulmonary and systemic immune systems.

2. Reduce inflammation of the trachea and bronchi.

3. Facilitate mucus expectoration.

4. Promote pulmonary blood circulation.

5. Identify and avoid allergens and airway irritants.

6. Speed up the cleansing process.

THERAPEUTIC RECOMMENDATIONS
FOODS

Eliminating dairy and wheat products during the infection helps to decrease mucus production and congestion. Primary foods specifically healing for bronchitis are black beans, azuki beans, mung beans, onions, garlic, yellow corn and blue corn (in such foods as the hot corn cereal atole or tortillas).

A healing broth prepared with dark leafy greens, parsley, carrots and/or squash is an excellent support. Use 1 cup up to 3 times a day. Sweet potatoes also are helpful. Secondary food choices include other legumes, whole grains, and fresh fruits and vegetables.

To liquify the mucus, plenty of warm fluids are needed. These may include medicinal herb teas, miso broth, vegetable bouillon, water with lemon and honey, and one part carrot or apricot juice mixed with one part pure water.

Sulfur dioxide, a common food additive in dried fruit, wines, beers, and used in salad bars, can act as an initiating factor in bronchial constriction and should be avoided. See Appendix E, p. 148.

BOTANICALS

Echinacea	4 parts	Take as a combined
Horehound	3 parts	extract, 30-50 drops every
Grindelia	3 parts	hour or two. Gargle and
Licorice	3 parts	swallow.

(formula continues on next page)

Yerba Mansa	2 parts
Black Cohosh	2 parts
Mullein	2 parts
Propolis	1 part

BASIS FOR THERAPEUTICS

Echinacea: Stimulates production, speed of maturation and aggressiveness of white blood cells toward intruders.

Horehound: Calms goblet cells' production of thick mucus while activating serous cells' production of thinner, more fluid mucus. Dilates the bronchioles.

Grindelia: Helps liquify mucus and facilitate its expectoration. Reduces dry spasmodic bronchial coughs.

Licorice: Reduces inflammation of the trachea and bronchi. Enhances absorption of other herbs.

Yerba Mansa: Tightens the connective tissues of the lungs. Stimulates lymph drainage. Speeds up removal of debris to initiate final repair.

Black Cohosh: Helps lessen irritation of the pulmonary nerves. Calms irritated bronchial mucus cells. Diminishes cough reflex. Increases thin mucus secretions in the bronchials.

Mullein: Is a mild sedative and anti-inflammatory for the lungs. Most beneficial at the beginning of infection, as it enhances moistening and early clearing of mucus.

Propolis: Discourages bacterial growth and stimulates respiratory circulation. Helps prevent edema and congestion in injured tissues. As with echinacea and yerba mansa, its caffeic acid content prevents further or secondary bacterial invasion.

SUPPLEMENTS

Vitamin A (Beta-carotene): 10,000-30,000 I.U. 3 times per day after meals for no more than five days, for a daily total of 10,000-90,000 I.U. per day. Not more than 15,000 I.U.

maximum if you are pregnant or trying to conceive. See ABOUT SUPPLEMENTS. See warning, p. 9.

A Good Multiple Vitamin and Mineral Formula: see p. 146. This one should have 200mcg. of selenium and the B vitamins as recommended.

Buffered vitamin C, Hypoallergenic: 1-6 gms. per day, taken hourly in 500 mg. doses.

Vitamin E: 600-800 I.U. after a meal.

Zinc gluconate lozenge: 15 mg. elemental, 5 times per day or 25 mg. 3 times per day after meals and at bedtime. Do not take on an empty stomach.

Iron: If symptoms of anemia or shortness of breath are present, 25 mg. with breakfast.

L-cysteine: 500 mg., 2 times per day, before breakfast and dinner

BASIS FOR THERAPEUTICS

Vitamin A: Strengthens bronchial cells and promotes their lubrication. Supports cell-mediated local lung defenses. Promotes white blood cell activity.

A Good Multiple Vitamin and Mineral Formula: the selenium reduces the effects of chemical sensitivity, especially vital in recurring bronchitis. The vitamin B complex's folic acid and B_{12} stimulate cell-mediated lung defenses. Along with selenium, vitamin C and L-cysteine, it is specifically useful for detoxification in acute bronchitis.

Vitamin C: Especially helpful in viral bronchitis or bronchitis related to toxic metal or chemical buildup. Promotes detoxification of heavy metals. Strengthens white blood cells.

Vitamin E: Particularly useful where there is a long-standing history of lung weakness. Enhances flexibility of lung tissue. Minimizes the toxic buildup of vitamin A.

Iron: Stimulates the immune cells' response within the

bronchi. Essential for cell-mediated immune system action.

Zinc: Increased amounts are used in the inflammatory state of this disorder. Stimulates T-cells action, helper cell production and thymulin (immune initiator) activity. Promotes active circulation of vitamin A.

L-cysteine: Liquifies mucus.

PREVENTION AND HEALING

Bed rest is suggested until fever goes away. Use moist heat on neck and upper chest.

Spring, summer and fall are the times to store up the energy needed to move through winter easily. Keep warm. Avoid chills. Satisfy your need to rest. If you are a smoker or live in an urban area, the suggested nutrients should be a part of your daily diet throughout the year.

Keep in mind that a good alternative to cheese is fresh fish. It is less congestive and is rich in protein and essential fatty acids which build lung membrane. Salmon is most highly recommended for this condition. It is a rich source of calcium, iron, B complex, selenium and vitamin E. (See ASTHMA, p. 95.)

Unresolved grief and sadness can have a debilitating effect upon the lungs. Being honest with yourself and those around you when a feeling comes up is one way to lighten the load on your lungs. An openness to new ideas and literally letting in fresh air in the form of regular deep breaths is healing.

VISUALIZATION

You are standing in a tall, cool, moist forest. You can feel the trees take in the breeze, expiring their wastes out fully and easily into the air.

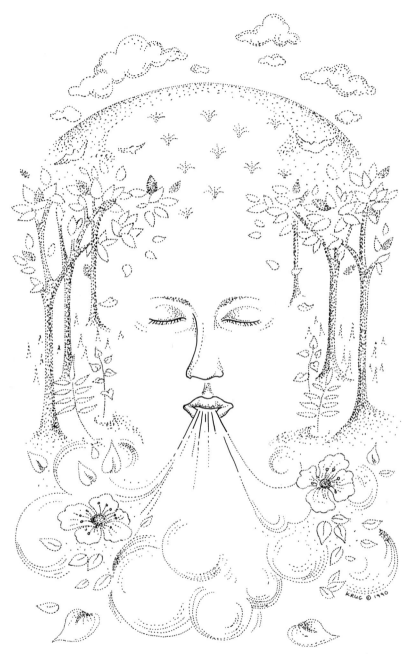

Creative Visualization

CHRONIC OBSTRUCTIVE PULMONARY DISEASE (C.O.P.D.)

DEFINITION

C.O.P.D. is a disorder which usually results in some permanent loss of breathing function. It manifests as airways obstruction. As it progresses there is increasing difficulty in exhaling fully. This disease classification includes chronic bronchitis, emphysema and chronic asthma.

DESCRIPTION

C.O.P.D. is the most common of the diseases of the lungs. It occurs most often in middle age. Cigarette smoking is the primary causal factor; another common cause being air pollution. The first major symptom usually is difficulty in breathing while walking, exercising or engaging in other physical exertion. A cough may be present for years before dyspnea appears. Examination usually reveals that only half the normal maximum breathing capacity remains. Chronic bronchitis and emphysema quite often are found together.

People in industrial areas that have cold, wet winters are more susceptible to C.O.P.D. In the United States, this disease is second only to heart disease as a cause of disability. Mortality rates for C.O.P.D. have been doubling every five years. Men are much more susceptible than women, presumably because of the greater length of time they have smoked and the greater number of cigarettes smoked per day. As more women choose to smoke, this gap is narrowing.

Respiratory tract infection will bring on a worsening of symptoms. Therefore prevention of infection is extremely important in controlling and healing C.O.P.D. C.O.P.D. can become your ally in maintaining maximum wellness.

BIOLOGICAL OVERVIEW

If C.O.P.D. progresses, there is a gradual loss of active lung tissue, including loss of the pulmonary capillaries. This will impede transportation of oxygen. To compensate for this, the body manufactures more red blood cells. This puts a burden on the right side of the heart and enlarges the right ventricle.

There is increasing obstruction of airflow when a breath is exhaled forcibly. Normal forceful expiration usually lasts about three to four seconds. In C.O.P.D., emptying time is at least five seconds. This is due to a loss of tissue and loss of elasticity of the lungs. If this stress continues long enough, it can lead to heart failure.

EMOTIONAL INFORMATION

Smoking can become a substitute for speaking up about the anger, hurt, fear or love you feel. These unexpressed feelings accumulate and create tension. Releasing a feeling can release tension in the chest. Talk about it. Breathe. Move. Write. Draw.

GUIDELINES FOR ACTION

1. Stop smoking (see p. 119).
2. Prevent or take care of any respiratory infection immediately.
3. Reduce inflammation.
4. Liquify and facilitate expectoration of sputum.
5. Alleviate bronchospasms by increasing dilation of bronchi.
6. Support and strengthen circulation from the heart to the lungs.
7. Learn as much as you can about the disease, its treatment and healing.

Foods rich in Vitamin A (Beta-Carotene)

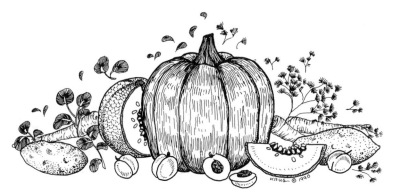

THERAPEUTIC RECOMMENDATIONS
FOODS

Two (1/2 C.) servings each day of any of the following foods will be extremely helpful in protecting the lungs: cantaloupe, apricots, sweet potato, pumpkin, winter squash, carrots and dark leafy greens such as kale, collards, mustard and turnip greens, parsley, and watercress. These foods are rich in beta-carotene.

BOTANICALS

Garlic (deodorized): 1 capsule 3 times per day with meals.

Chlorophyll concentrate: 20 drops 2 or 3 times per day immediately before meals.

Mullein	6 parts	Take as a combined extract
Coltsfoot	4 parts	20-30 drops 3 times per
Elecampane	4 parts	day: mid-morning, mid
Grindelia	3 parts	afternoon, and evening
Echinacea	3 parts	(preferably one hour
Inmortal	3 parts	before sleep).
Passion flower	2 parts	
Osha	2 parts	
Lobelia	1 part	
Yerba Santa	1 part	
Blood root	1 part	

Garlic: Increases resistance to bacterial infection, including staphylococcus and streptococcus. Combats fungus infections, including Candida albicans. Prevents clumping of lymphocytes, reducing the spread of viral disease.

Chlorophyll: Increases circulation of oxygen by strengthening red blood cell oxygen-binding capacity.

Mullein: Reduces inflammation of respiratory tissues. Tones mucous membranes. Facilitates expectoration. Decreases bronchospasms. Ideal for long term management of lung problems.

Coltsfoot: Stabilizes mast cells' secretion of histamine (inflammatory compounds). Specific for C.O.P.D. which is aggravated by allergies. Soothes irritation of bronchial mucosa.

Elecampane: Soothes and calms coughs. Its antimicrobial action prevents infections.

Grindelia: Calms rapid heartbeat. Relaxes smooth muscles of bronchi, dilating them. Liquifies thick mucus. Stimulates expectoration of sputum. Stimulates repair of damaged lung tissues.

Echinacea: Promotes lung defenses. Prevents lung infection. The dosage of this herb (as a single extract) may be increased at the onset of infection.

Inmortal: Supports the right side of the heart. Stimulates lymph drainage from the lungs. Is a mild bronchial dilator.

Passion flower: Supports respiratory center in the brain stem. Helps calm anxiety related to breathing.

Osha: Stimulates production of thin mucus. Acts as a bronchial dilator. Stimulates cilia's clearance of sputum.

Lobelia: Stops spasms of the respiratory system. Alleviates irritability of the pulmonary nervous system.

Yerba Santa: Arrests excessive mucous secretions.

Blood Root: Increases blood flow through the lungs.

SUPPLEMENTS

Beta-carotene: 10,000-25,000 I.U. once per day after a meal. See warning p. 9.

B-Complex: once per day after meals.

Vitamin C: 1,000 mg. once per day after a meal.

Vitamin E: 600-1,000 I.U. once per day after a meal. See warning p. 8.

Selenium: 200 mcg. once per day after a meal.

Zinc gluconate: A minimum of 15 mg. per day, and up to 50 mg. per day for heavy smokers. Once per day after a meal.

L-Cysteine: 500 mg. 2 times per day before meals.

Linseed Oil, capsules or liquid: 2,000 mg. 2 times per day after meals.

BASIS OF THERAPEUTICS

Beta-carotene: Increases macrophage immune activity. Beta-carotene gives the best results when derived directly from foods. Stimulates T- cells and T helper cells which are key immune system components. Reduces the risk of infection by bacteria or fungi.

B complex: Detoxifies chemicals from smoking (past and present). B6 helps eliminate cadmium, a toxin found in cigarettes. Improves oxygen transport and circulation. Strengthens immune system function, thereby preventing infections.

Vitamin C: Promotes production of interferon, which protects against viral infections. Strengthens the white blood cells.

Vitamin E: Improves elasticity and flexibility of the lungs, thus increasing oxygen transport and enhancing ease of breathing. Decreases viscosity of the blood. Allergies to vitamin E in supplement form may occur.

Selenium: A key nutrient. Strengthens lung tissue. Minimizes damage from smoke of all types. Strengthens the heart muscle. Strengthens the immune function and (with vitamins A, E and C) reduces the risk of lung cancer. Zinc: Promotes the circulation of beta-carotene in the blood. Detoxifies cadmium from tobacco smoke and other pollutants.

L-cysteine: Liquifies mucus. Protects the lungs against smoke damage of all kinds. Specifically protects the alveoli by stimulating macrophage activity, thereby reducing the risk of infection.

Linseed Oil: Its essential fatty acids promote healthy lubrication of lung membrane tissue.

PREVENTION AND HEALING

1. Breathing exercises (See Appendix A, p. 128.)

2. Walking at a good pace. Start with an amount of time that is comfortable for you and work up to 1/2 hour a day.

3. Siberian Ginseng: 15-20 drops twice per day before meals. This herb is an adaptogen.

Rapid resolution of any respiratory infection is the most important action in managing C.O.P.D., especially chronic bronchitis. Minimizing chemical exposure is the second highest priority. Stopping smoking addresses both priorities. Smoking seriously depletes the immune strengtheners: vitamin A, vitamin C, selenium and zinc. Seventy-five per cent of smokers are chemically sensitive to tobacco and its components. Minimizing exposure to smoke and other contaminants gives the lungs a chance to heal.

VISUALIZATION

Imagine a healthy vibrant tree swaying in a gentle breeze. This tree becomes your lungs. You sense an aliveness, rooted in joy, that heals you.

EMPHYSEMA

Note: The following text is directed to those who are dealing primarily with emphysema. To get the fullest picture
of this condition, please read the section on CHRONIC
OBSTRUCTIVE PULMONARY DISEASE, p. 74.

DEFINITION
Emphysema is a C.O.P.D. characterized by an increase
in size of the air spaces of the lungs. Walls of air sacs and
respiratory bronchioles are destroyed.

DESCRIPTION
Emphysema occurs most frequently in people who
smoke. Symptoms, which usually do not appear until
mid-life (fiftyish), include: shortness of breath, chronic
cough and expectoration of thick mucoid sputum. Respiration usually is abnormally rapid and there is often the
sensation of not getting enough air. As the person strains
to get sufficient air, the diaphram flattens and the space
behind the sternum becomes enlarged. Unless they are
cared for promptly, the lungs lose their elasticity.

BIOLOGICAL OVERVIEW
The lungs are structured in such a way as to provide
maximum surface area in the least space possible. If all the
air sacs and respiratory tubes were fully extended, their
surface area would measure approximately 70 square
yards. This is about the size of a tennis court.

The adult lung contains some 300 million alveoli. Each
of these alveoli is surrounded by an intricate blood supply system designed to facilitate oxygen/carbon dioxide
exchange. In emphysema, alveoli are destroyed and larger
spaces are created in the lungs. This process decreases the
number of blood capillaries in the lungs and diminishes
the total surface area available for gas exchange. If this
process continues unchecked, the airways can begin to

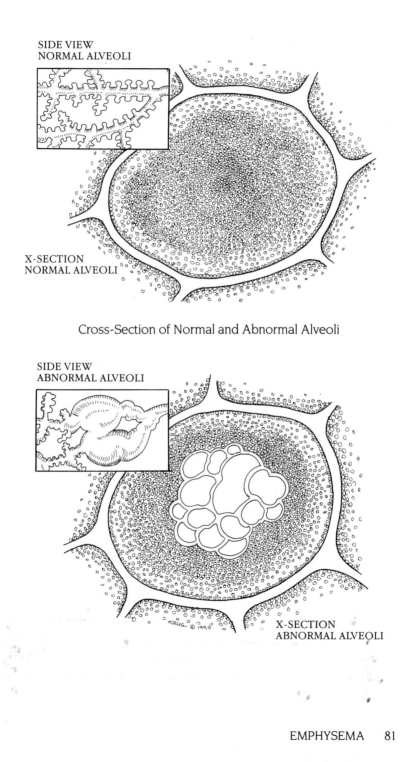

SIDE VIEW
NORMAL ALVEOLI

X-SECTION
NORMAL ALVEOLI

Cross-Section of Normal and Abnormal Alveoli

SIDE VIEW
ABNORMAL ALVEOLI

X-SECTION
ABNORMAL ALVEOLI

collapse on expiration. It is critical to stop degeneration, thus protecting proper gas exchange, blood flow and lymphatic function. Even if much tissue has been destroyed before action is taken, it is possible to learn to maximize lung efficiency and still lead a full, productive life.

In 15 per cent of all cases, a genetic deficit of the enzyme alpha I antitrypsin contributes to emphysema. A simple medical test will tell you if you have this deficiency.

EMOTIONAL INFORMATION

Emphysema frequently relates to a reluctance to share feelings, a holding in of emotions. There may be a tendency to hide who you really are, or assume that you are unimportant in the larger scheme of things. Often you may set aside and negate your many small needs and desires. Being willing to trust your feelings and to express them are vital in breaking this pattern.

GUIDELINES FOR ACTION

1. See C.O.P.D. p. 75.

2. Stop smoking.

3. Increase oxygen intake, ventilation and blood circulation through the lungs.

4. Slow down or stop alveoli destruction.

5. Strengthen and use abdominal muscles for active exhalation (see Appendix A, p. 128).

THERAPEUTICS RECOMMENDATIONS

See C.O.P.D., p. 76 The following are supplementary recommendations.

FOODS

Selenium-rich foods are especially useful for smokers and ex-smokers: fresh and canned salmon, shrimp, tuna, oysters, turkey, organic kidney meats, brazil nuts, sunflower seeds, cracked wheat bread, whole wheat cereals, molasses. One to two servings per day of the above foods provide 60 mcg. of selenium per 100 gm. serving.

Foods abundant in vitamin A and silica help maintain and repair lung membranes. Vitamin A also is needed in greater amounts by smokers and ex-smokers. Foods high in vitamin A include carrots, broccoli, cantaloupe, dark leafy greens, yams, pumpkin, acorn squash, apricots, and spirulina. Silica-rich foods include oatmeal, string beans, onions, garlic and leeks.

Avoiding dairy foods can reduce lung congestion. If there is a long history of use of antibiotics or steroid sprays, a yeast-free diet may be necessary. (See FUNGAL RESPIRATORY INFECTIONS., p. 102.)

Fresh and dried ginger, as a tea and added to foods, liquify mucus. Ginger also aids bowel elimination.

BASIS OF THERAPEUTICS

Selenium-rich foods strengthen lung and heart tissue. They support the immune system and detoxify tobacco smoke waste products.

Foods containing vitamin A maintain and rebuild mucous membranes.

Silica-rich foods help stabilize and strengthen lung septa (alveolar walls).

For further suggestions about foods, see CHRONIC BRONCHITIS, p. 88.

BOTANICALS

See C.O.P.D. recommendations and add the following:

Horsetail	3 parts	20-30 drops not more than
Horehound	2 parts	5 times per day.
Plantain	2 parts	
Lungwort	2 parts	

BASIS OF THERAPEUTICS

Horsetail: Is rich in silica. Helps stabilize and strengthen lung septa (alveolar walls).

Horehound: An alveolar vasodilator. Also a very useful expectorant.

Plantain: Helps reduce irritation of the respiratory membranes. Soothing in chronic emphysema.

Lungwort: Decreases excess mucous production. Relaxes the smooth muscles of the bronchi. Facilitates expectoration.

SUPPLEMENTS

See C.O.P.D. recommendations, p. 78.

PREVENTION AND HEALING:

Stop smoking. This is absolutely essential if you are going to heal yourself. Chemical or cadmium exposure can be another cause of the disorder. Avoiding this, if it is present, is equally important. Living in a city or other air-polluted region increases stress to the lungs. Relocation to a non-industrial area is recommended, if this is possible.

Since inhalation is favored in emphysema, it is important to encourage exhalation. Slow walking, gradually building up time and distance, is helpful. Singing, whistling, or playing an instrument like a horn, flute or tin whistle, also promotes full expiration of air. These activities strengthen the bronchioles and keep them open.

It is vital to stop stressing the lungs.

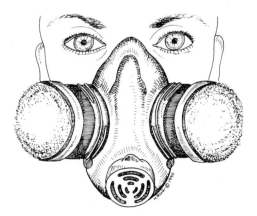

Elevate the foot of the bed 12-22 degrees to ease and enhance the functioning of the diaphragm for abdominal breathing during sleep.

Sometimes silver-mercury (amalgam) dental fillings are a secondary debilitating stress on the system. They increase nutritional needs for selenium and vitamins E, C and B-complex.

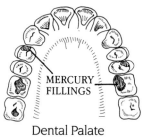

Dental Palate

Preventing infections with the help of the foods and herbs described above will speed up your healing and lengthen your lifespan.

VISUALIZATION

You are seeing trees opening thousands upon thousands of healthy vibrant leaves. Each tree is constantly replenishing itself with new leaves. Feel the leaves gently swaying in the breeze.

NOTES

CHRONIC BRONCHITIS

Note: The following text is directed to those who are dealing primarily with chronic bronchitis. To get the fullest picture of this condition, see CHRONIC OBSTRUCTIVE PULMONARY DISEASE, p. 74.

DEFINITION

Chronic bronchitis usually is caused by prolonged exposure to bronchial irritants (e.g., substances released in tobacco smoke. This disorder is specifically diagnosed only after a productive cough has been present three months of the year for at least three consecutive years.

DESCRIPTION

Chronic bronchitis is characterized by a chronic productive cough. Sputum is abundant and may plug the smaller bronchioles. Without proper care, recurrent infections are common. This disorder is most often associated with cigarette smoking and is found in 20 per cent of adult males. It is most commonly diagnosed in people in their late 40s.

BIOLOGICAL OVERVIEW

The cough of chronic bronchitis results from an effort of the lungs to improve mucus-clearing capacity. To meet attack from smoke or other irritants, the lungs increase the number of thick mucus secreting cells in the bronchial walls. This results in an increase in thickness of these walls which hinders oxygen exchange and breath. The new cells produce an excessive amount of sputum. When the cilia, in charge of removing sputum, cannot meet the increased demand, sputum begins to accumulate. If this condition persists for some months, the small airways become inflamed and can slowly fill with unexpelled materials. Bacteria, viruses and fungi then find it easier to invade the lungs and infections may become habitual. An accumulation of carbon dioxide and a deficient supply of oxygen may complicate this condition. In an effort to increase gas exchange, the heart must work harder to increase blood flow through the lungs.

It is extremely important to support the body in arresting a possible degeneration of the lungs and in stimulating their repair.

EMOTIONAL INFORMATION

There is a tendency for congestion, for potentially toxic feelings to accumulate as wastes. Often the individual is a deeply feeling person who thinks that expressing emotion is not in keeping with her/his self-image. Chronic bronchitis may signal a need to express anger in a positive and creative way. The need to consistently acknowledge feelings and allow them to move is important. Do intense physical exercise (when you are well). Take action on "gut" feelings. These will help release long-term congestion.

GUIDELINES FOR ACTION

1. Decrease bronchial tube inflammation.

2. See also C.O.P.D., p. 75.

THERAPEUTIC RECOMMENDATIONS
FOODS

A diet rich in nourishing foods is extremely important in healing chronic bronchitis. Often there is an underlying family history of food sensitivity, particularly if celiac disease, stomach problems, osteoarthritis, premature graying, cancer, lupus, leukemia, Alzheimer's or depression have been present in the family. In such cases, there frequently is a genetic correlation with grain and/or dairy foods sensitivity.

Eliminating all dairy and wheat products for ten days is highly recommended. These include butter, milk, cheese, ice cream, yogurt, sour cream, whipping cream, milk fats, milk proteins, cream sauces, whey; white flour, whole wheat flour, wheat bran, wheat germ, pasta (including spinach, artichoke and tomato pastas, which contain wheat), and bread, tortillas, crackers and muffins made with wheat flour.

Particularly in our culture where these foods are served at every meal, this can be very difficult to do. Yet many people have found so striking a relief of symptoms from forgoing them that they are willing to make the effort.

Rye, oats and barley sometimes cause allergic reactions. Other grains and grain products, such as the following, may be substituted: corn, rice, cornmeal, corn tortillas, rice flour, rice bread, rice cakes, rice crackers and buckwheat. Soba, a pasta made entirely from buckwheat, is an alternative to wheat pasta. Occasionally there may be an allergic reaction to one of these grains, as well, which may manifest as sinus stuffiness, congestion, fatigue, aching joints or restless sleep. In such cases, after isolating the offender by a process of elimination, it too should be avoided.

Eggs are usually an acceptable food in chronic bronchitis. Nut milk, coconut milk and/or rice milk may be substituted for cow's milk. Sometimes goat's milk is tolerated when cow's milk is not. Lentils and soy products are usually good protein substitutes and rich in molybdenum, although they may cause allergic reactions in some individuals. The allergy symptoms listed above can tip you off.

Sulfites, metabisulfites, bisulfites and sulfur dioxide are commonly used in processed and restaurant foods. These

Foods Which May
Contain Sulfites

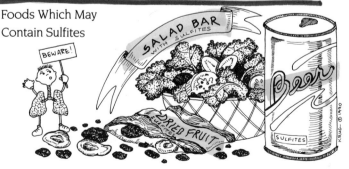

can set off bronchial constriction when there is no infection present and therefore should be scrupulously avoided. (See Appendix E, p. 148.)

BOTANICALS

Follow C.O.P.D. recommendations in addition to the following formula:

Nettles	3 parts	Take as a liquid herbal
Osha	2 parts	extract 10 drops, 3 times
Horehound	2 parts	per day.
Plaintain	2 parts	
Ma Huang	2 parts	
Licorice	1 part	

BASIS OF THERAPEUTICS

Nettles: Decrease allergic reactions. Prevent excessive production of mucus. Decrease inflammation of the airways.

Osha: Helps to liquify the mucus and to remove it from the lung.

Horehound: Relaxes smooth muscles of the bronchi. Helps increase sputum expectoration. Promotes action of Osha.

Plantain: Provides relief from coughing, pain, irritation and wheezing. It also is a good expectorant.

Ma Huang: Dilates the bronchioles. Reduces allergic reactions. (See Warning p. 5.)

Licorice: Enhances the action of other herbs. An anti-inflammatory.

SUPPLEMENTS

Follow C.O.P.D. recommendations in addition to:

Pantothenic acid: 250-500 mg.: 1 to 3 times per day, after meals.

Vitamin C: An additional 500-2,000 mg. (1,500-3,000 mg. total daily) in 500-1,000 mg. doses, 3 times per day after meals.

B-Complex: A double dose 2 times per day after meals as recommended (see C.O.P.D., p. 78.)

Molybdenum: 50-100 mcg., once a day after a meal.

BASIS OF THERAPEUTICS

Pantothenic Acid: Prevents attacks of bronchitis. Strengthens the sinus tissue. Acts as a natural anti-histamine by preventing and minimizing upper respiratory infections and allergic reactions to pollens. May protect against sulfur dioxide poisoning.

Vitamin C: Reduces sulfite damage.

B-Complex: B1, B2 and folic acid are depleted by toxic exposure to sulfites. B12 can prevent toxic reactions to metabisulfite.

Molybdenum: Activates sulfite oxidase, the enzyme which detoxifies poisonous sulfite into non-toxic sulfate.

PREVENTION AND HEALING

Clean air, exercise, plenty of fluids and a chemical-, drug- and tobacco-free environment are most important in preventing chronic bronchitis.

VISUALIZATION

Imagine you are in an irritating situation. Let yourself say whatever you feel about this. Then imagine you are gently stroking your chest, taking in cool soothing air with every stroke.

ASTHMA

Note: To get the fullest picture of this condition, please read the section on CHRONIC OBSTRUCTIVE PULMONARY DISEASE, p. 74. The following text is directed to those who are dealing primarily with asthma.

DEFINITION

Asthma, a chronic obstructive pulmonary disease, is a reversible airways obstruction not caused by any other disease. It is characterized by an increased responsiveness of the airways (i.e., the bronchial tubes close). With proper care, there is no need for asthma to become a permanent debilitating condition.

DESCRIPTION

Common symptoms of asthma include difficulty in breathing, coughing, wheezing, use of accessory muscles to facilitate breathing, apprehension, fast beating heart (up to 120 beats per minute), flaring nostrils and increasing symptoms of respiratory distress. Tightness of chest and thick and tenacious production of mucus are also seen. The underlying mechanisms which create attacks of sudden wheezing are not fully understood.

Asthma affects approximately 4 percent of the American population (about 9 million people). Up to 7 percent of Americans will experience asthma at one time or another during their lifetime. It occurs most frequently in children and young adults and is the most common cause of school absence and hospital admission in children. *Fifty to seventy percent of children outgrow the disease.*

Confirmed contributory factors are: genetic predisposition; viral respiratory infection; emotional upset; inhalation of cold air, fresh paint, tobacco smoke, chemical fumes and other irritants; exposure to specific allergens (foods, liquids or fabrics); and such non-specific factors as change in temperature. A family history of asthma or allergies, such as eczema, is found in about half of asthmatics.

Asthma is divided in two broad categories:

(a) Extrinsic or allergic asthma: It is brought on when the person comes in contact with allergens—airborne pollens and molds, animal danders, foods, drugs and house dust. These symptoms are IgE mediated: IgE or Immunoglobulin E is an antibody produced by the cells lining the respiratory and intestinal tracts. In asthmatics, when an allergen enters the respiratory tract, an allergen IgE antibody reaction takes place. This leads to the allergic reaction. As a result, mast cells will secrete "Slow Releasing Substance of Anaphylaxsis" and other inflammatory compounds. SRS-A causes spasms of bronchiole tubes. Ten to twenty percent of the adult asthmatic population is affected by this kind of asthma.

(b) Intrinsic asthma: In this condition, asthma occurs in people not identified, by history or tests, as suffering from allergies. The precipitating causes may be, for example, infections, irritants or emotional factors.

Status asthmaticus describes a prolonged and potentially dangerous attack of very severe asthma.

BIOLOGICAL OVERVIEW

Asthma usually manifests as three sets of physical changes:

(a) Bronchospasms may develop to the point where considerable obstruction occurs.

(b) Bronchial walls become inflamed and swell up. This creates further narrowing of airways.

(c) Mucus glands produce a thick tenacious mucus.

All of these changes lead to hyperinflation of the lungs because inhaling is easier than exhaling. Over a short period of time air exchange problems and increasingly labored respiration develops. This breathing problem often spontaneously disappears in a matter of minutes.

Asthma seems to be created by an imbalance in the relative functions of the sympathetic and parasympathetic nervous systems as they relate to the lungs. The sympathetic nervous system is stimulated by adrenal gland secretions, especially epinephrine and norepinephrine. This system is often deficient in asthma. Normally, these hormones calm mast cell inflammatory response and relax bronchial muscles. The parasympathetic nervous system, by means of the vagus nerve, has an opposite action. It stimulates inflammation and bronchial constriction and thereby aggravates this condition. The parasympathetic nervous system is often overactive in asthma.

Balance must be restored by means of proper adrenal gland functioning. Subclinical adrenal gland deficiency generally is not recognized by the medical profession. Yet this is frequently an underlying cause of asthma.

EMOTIONAL INFORMATION

Asthma is, in essence, an excessive response to a stimuli. This may indicate harboring of repressed fear or anger. Every little challenge in life can be seen as a gigantic one, so that all alarms are sounded and all resources are channelled toward the challenge.

Asthma can offer an opportunity to take whatever space you need for yourself, emotionally as well as physically. It is important to feel your own strength directly. Begin to acknowledge the strengths you have inside; list them, speak them out loud.

GUIDELINES FOR ACTION

If you smoke, stop.

In acute attack:

If major: Seek immediate help. Go see your doctor or go to the emergency room of a hospital.

If minor:

1. dilate the bronchioles

2. facilitate expectoration

3. reduce inflammation of lung tissues.

For long-term healing:

1. support adrenal glands

2. stabilize mast cells throughout the body

3. decrease stress level

4. increase body's resistance to challenges.

THERAPEUTIC RECOMMENDATIONS

FOODS

Foods can trigger an asthmatic attack, particularly in children. Cow's milk, yeast, cheese, fish, nuts, chocolate, wheat, eggs, shellfish, tomatoes and other foods of the nightshade family (for example eggplant and potatoes) are potential offenders. High-salicylate foods can aggravate 10-20% of asthmatics (see Appendix D, p. 149.) Aspirin, food colorings and monosodium glutomate (MSG) can initiate an episode. Avoid processed and salted foods as much as possible.

Flaxseed and linseed oils, and salmon, if tolerated, are rich in essential fatty acids. These can be useful long-term promoters of bronchial relaxation. Red meat can have the opposite effect, stimulating constriction. Therefore it should be eaten no more than once or twice a week.

If you or your child have been using steroids for some time, there are special nutritional considerations. You will particularly need to balance your blood sugar, keep your potassium levels up and reduce your intake of salt. Small frequent meals and protein snacks (beans, chicken, turkey) can be helpful. Most fruits, vegetables, and whole grains are high-potassium foods, especially avocados, carrots (best taken in the high potency form of carrot juice) and bananas. Mineral repletion may be necessary, as corticosteroids deplete the body of calcium, magnesium and zinc.

See also Foods, CHRONIC BRONCHITIS, p. 88.

BOTANICALS

Siberian Ginseng: 20 drops, twice a day for six months or longer.

Acute Phase

Ma Huang	6 parts	Take as a combined extract
Grindelia	5 parts	20 -40 drops every 2 hours
Licorice	4 parts	during acute attacks. Dur-
Osha	4 parts	ing remission use C.O.P.D
Pleurisy Root	3 parts	formula.
Lobelia	1 part	

Long Term Healing

Coltsfoot	2 parts	Take as a combined extract
Nettles	2 parts	20 drops 3 times per day
Elecampane	1 part	between meals. Must be
Passion flower	1 part	taken on a long-term basis
		to achieve desired results.

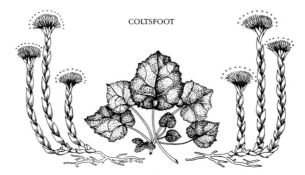

COLTSFOOT

BASIS OF THERAPEUTICS

Siberian Ginseng: Is an adaptogen—a substance which increases the capacity of the body to adapt to a wide range of biological, chemical and other physical stresses.

Ma Huang: Stimulates the sympathetic nervous system to produce a relaxation of the smooth muscles of the respiratory system. Assists full broncho-dilation.

Grindelia: Liquifies thick mucus. Reduces excess production of mucus.

Licorice: Supports the adrenals. Enhances the actions of other herbs. An excellent anti-inflammatory.

Osha: Acts as a broncho-dilator. Stimulates the diaphragm, thus producing deep breathing. Softens mucus and increases cilia motility promoting the clearance of mucus.

Pleurisy Root: Decreases broncho-pulmonic inflammation. Eases pain between the ribs and along the sternum. Most helpful when the cough is dry and mucus is scant.

Lobelia: A potent herb. Stops spasms of the bronchioles. A respiratory stimulant. SEE WARNING, p. 6.

Coltsfoot: Helps stabilize mast cells, preventing their excessive release of Slow Releasing Substance of Anaphylasis.

Nettles: Has the same action as coltsfoot.

Elecampane: Prevents spasms of the bronchioles. Maintains proper fluidity of lung secretions.

Passion Flower: Prevents excess irritability of the bronchioles.

SUPPLEMENTS

Note: Children should take the lowest recommended dose, unless otherwise recommended by a qualified health practitioner.

In addition to C.O.P.D. recommendations, take:

Vitamin B_6: 50-100 mg. once per day after breakfast.

Pantothenic Acid: 100-500 mg. 3 times per day after meals.

Vitamin C: 10,000 mg. maximum taken in divided mg. doses throughout the day.

B-complex: two capsules per day after meals.

L-cysteine: 500 mg. 2-3 times per day with two cups of fluids before meals.

L-tyrosine: 250-500 mg. twice per day before meals.

Linseed or flax oil: 1,000-5,000 mg. once a day with meals.

Hydrochloric acid and/or pancreatin: one capsule after a large meal.

Bioflavonoids: 1,000 mg., 1-3 times per day.

BASIS OF THERAPEUTICS

Vitamin B$_6$: Specifically helpful for asthma, presumably by catalyzing neurohormonal mediator response in the lung tissue. Counteracts MSG poisoning.

Pantothenic acid: An excellent promoter of adrenal hormone production of epinephrine and norepinephrine. Strengthens sinus tissue. Has an antihistaminic action.

Vitamin C: Like pantothenic acid, stimulates antihistamine response. With B-complex, used in the production of epinephrine and nor-epinephrine which reduce bronchial constriction. Strengthens adrenals and therefore is essential especially if steroids have been or are in use.

B complex: Folic acid works with tyrosine to reduce bronchial constriction through activation of norepinephrine and epinephrine.

L-cysteine: See C.O.P.D., p. 79.

L-tyrosine: Stimulates production of epinephrine and noropinephrine, thereby helping to prevent bronchial constriction.

Linseed or flaxseed oils: Rich in Omega-3 linolenic acid. This essential fatty acid stimulates production of prostaglandin E, which dilates the bronchioles and calms inflammation. May stabilize mast cells.

Hydrochloric acid and/or pancreatin: Most useful if asthma attacks are related to food sensitivity. These help break down food proteins most completely, thereby minimizing allergic reactions.

Bioflavonoids: Potent antihistamines.

Normal stress is healthy and stimulating and it is, impractical to attempt to eliminate all stress from our lives. Asthmatics, however, frequently live on the edge of an acute and incapacitating distress precipitated by such elements as chemicals, dust, molds, pet dander, allergenic foods, emotional challenges, and fatigue. The asthmatic's key to the restoration of free breathing is to enlarge the cushion between her/him and acute stress. To do this, one needs to support the adrenals, minimize allergen and chemical exposure, enhance tolerance and strength, and create enough "space to breathe."

Enhancing tolerance means raising the distress threshold, so that stress does not immediately precipitate an asthma attack. Physically, tolerance can be strengthened by using the recommended foods, herbs and supplements. Mentally and emotionally, tolerance is strengthened through the individual's greater awareness of how he/she contributes to the stress level. Meditation can be very useful in this process.

Many sufferers from childhood asthma find that the asthma clears when they leave home. Possibly they are leaving behind such irritating substances as pet dander and mold. However, a common factor in this healing is the independent creation of new emotional space. Adults of more mature years also can affect a healing by taking similar action or measures. It is important for people with asthma to define physical and emotional boundaries in their lives.

Withdrawing from the use of inhalers and other medications is a challenge for many asthmatics, but it can be done.

However, DON'T TRY TO DO THIS ALONE. Don't stop any of these medications cold turkey. Seek the guidance and support of a physician who is willing to monitor a gradual reduction of the amounts and frequency of use of your medication. Under the supervision of such a physician, these general guidelines may be followed:

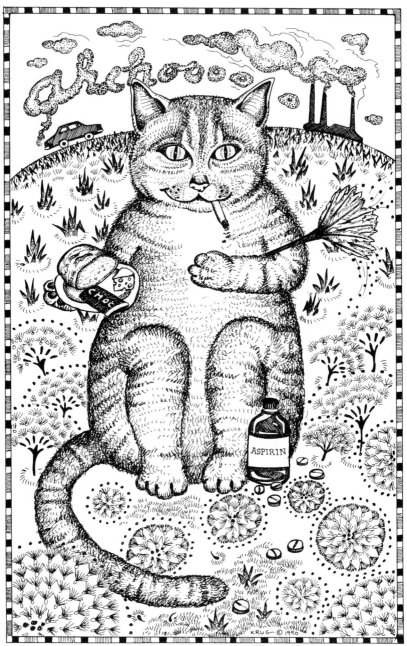

Most Common Allergens

1. Withdraw from one medicine at a time, gradually reducing the dosage. Decrease it by the smallest amount that is pragmatically possible. This may require breaking tablets into halves or quarters, or getting a prescription for a smaller dosage of the medicine.

2. Wait one week at the new level of medicine before reducing it further.

3. Wait until one medicine has been completely eliminated before starting to withdraw from the next.

4. If asthma symptoms develop or worsen, go back to the previous level of dosage until the symptoms clear. Wait one week, and then continue the tapering off process as outlined above.

If you are cutting down on antihistamines, increasing your intake of vitamin C, bioflavonoids and pantothenic acid will be helpful. These act as natural antihistamines, stimulating your cells' ability to process and cleanse the inflammatory histamines.

As you cut down on cromolyn and other inhalers, coltsfoot (5 times a day) and L-cysteine (3 times a day) may be used to help keep your lungs clear and breathing freely. You also may find it helpful during this process to gradually increase the distance between the inhaler spray and your mouth. Passion flower can be especially useful in calming tension related to changing medicinal schedules. These herbs and nutrients strengthen the tissues as they provide support. They can be discontinued gradually within three months to two years after you have successfully withdrawn the medications.

VISUALIZATION

You are in a large clear open space. You have all the room that you need. You can invite anyone you like into your space, and you can ask anyone to leave it. Feel the strength of this space inside you.

FUNGAL RESPIRATORY INFECTIONS

DEFINITION

Fungal respiratory infections include pneumonia, bronchitis and any other respiratory infection initiated by a fungus. They often occur as a result of antibiotic therapy for another infection.

DESCRIPTION

There are two kinds of fungal respiratory infections. (a) In primary infection, which is relatively rare, the inhalation of specific soil fungi causes such diseases as coccidioidomycosis, histoplasmosis, spirotrichosis, cryptococcosis, or North American blastomycosis. Farmers, miners and archaeologists in certain geographic regions are at greater risk. These diseases may initially present themselves as respiratory problems. In other cases, respiratory difficulties develop sometime after the fungal infection is contracted. Medical attention should be sought immediately. (b) Secondary or opportunistic infection is much more common, and is particularly responsive to nutritional and botanical therapies. At its mildest the infection may manifest as a slight itching in the throat or nasal passages and, at its most severe, as a full-blown pneumonia. Possible symptoms include chronic nasal congestion, chronic cough, repeated ear infections, nose, throat and bronchial infections, and pervasive fatigue. The symptoms often are aggravated by sweets, alcohol, bread, unrecognized food sensitivities, and a wide variety of chemicals, either inhaled or ingested, and damp weather. Frequently the infection arises during or after treatment with antibiotics or steroids, or with the use of estrogens.

These infections are a direct indication of depleted physical resources. They also can manifest during times of changing physiologic function, such as pregnancy, obesity and diabetic acidosis.

Among the infecting organisms are Candida albicans, Cryptococcus, and Nocardia, to name a few. Fatigue, depression, indigestion, mood swings, skin rashes, headaches, and lowered sex drive can be secondary symptoms of the infection. Low-grade fungal infections elsewhere in the body can alert you to the possibility of a low-grade chronic fungal respiratory infection. These can be infections under the fingernails or toenails, athlete's foot, vaginitis or thrush.

In both types of fungal infection, healing will be faster if other underlying physical imbalances and infections are identified and treated first.

BIOLOGICAL OVERVIEW

Fungi are plant-like organisms. They live on decaying or dead matter (as saprophytes) or at the expense of their host (as parasites). They are important recyclers of organic wastes, and some are normal elements of human microflora. There are some 100,000 to 200,000 known species of fungi. One hundred of these are common to humans, and fewer than a dozen will produce diseases in man.

Most fungi that are capable of causing disease in humans exist in spore or tissue forms. The fungal spore is stable in hostile environments. In tissue form, it eats, reproduces, and grows. These fungi can then become so populous that they cause infections, called mycoses, usually when there are few predators or competitors of fungi present.

Normally bacteria compete with fungi for living space in humans. If bacteria are wiped out, as they are in broad-spectrum antibiotic use, the fungi can proliferate unchecked.

Normally fungi are held in check by the presence of friendly bacteria and healthy immune and digestive function. A fungal infection lets you know there is an imbalance in the body's microbial population. Mycoses are strong indicators that the body needs some deep healing. The goal of treatment is to restore the immunological (and, in some cases, digestive) strength of the body and to re-establish normal microbial balance.

EMOTIONAL INFORMATION

There can be a tendency to let hurt, anger, resentment or mistrust "eat" at you. Or you may gnaw away at yourself, rerunning painful old experiences of abuse or mistreatment. This must be stopped. Catch yourself in these habitual painful patterns. Begin to introduce fresh thoughts: "I am healing." "I am developing healthy relationships." "I am taking care of myself." Allowing repetition of the old hopeless thoughts will bog you down even more deeply.

Ignoring your physical health and well-being (or lack thereof) is another pattern which can be conducive to fungal infections.. In such cases, a fungal respiratory infection alerts you to the true condition of your body and its need for healing.

GUIDELINES FOR ACTION

1. With the assistance of your physician, re-evaluate the use of antibiotics, immunosuppressive drugs, corticosteroids, and/or estrogens. If possible, gradually but completely eliminate these.

2. Stop the growth of the fungi.

3. Stimulate the immune and digestive systems.

4. Treat the underlying weak areas.

5. Re-establish healthy microbial balance.

6. Rebuild mucous membranes, especially of the respiratory tract.

7. Continue treatment long enough (6 months minimum) to insure that the fungal infection truly has been eliminated.

THERAPEUTIC RECOMMENDATIONS
FOODS

Diet is extremely important in freeing oneself of excess fungus/yeast. Foods which should absolutely be avoided include: alcohol; sugar; yeasted breads, rolls and crackers; hard cheeses; concentrated sweets like dried fruits; fried foods; preservatives; chemicals; and moldy foods (like blue cheese, tempeh and/or spoiled foods). It will be helpful to avoid such foods as vinegar and other fermented foods, tofu, smoked and processed meats like hot dogs and cold cuts, milk, malted products, fruit juices, herb teas, melons (especially cantaloupes), peanuts, pistachios and any left-overs.

Lest you wonder what you can eat on a strict yeast-free diet, these are fine: whole grains, oatmeal, rice, wheat, millet, corn, barley, quinoa, amaranth, buckwheat, unyeasted crackers, matzo, tortillas, rice cakes, unsweetened quick breads, biscuits and muffins; nuts and seeds like almonds, sunflower seeds, walnuts, filberts, brazil nuts, pecans, pumpkin seeds, cashews, sesame seeds, oils and butter; fresh fish, poultry and unprocessed meats; just about any vegetable including avocado, asparagus, artichoke, beets, broccoli, brussels sprouts, garlic, onions, turnips, cabbage, etc.; all beans and peas; water and mineral water and fresh lemon juice.

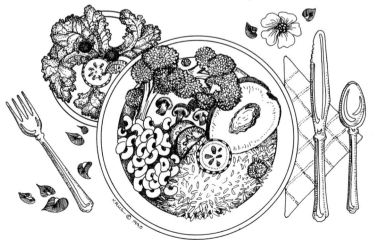

A moderate yeast-free diet also could include plain yogurt, cottage cheese, fresh fruit, fresh squeezed fruit juice, milk (in some cases), and some well-refrigerated or frozen left-overs.

Focus on high-quality protein foods and vegetables. Limit intake of carbohydrates and starchy snacks, like chips, especially eaten alone. More than one or two pieces of fresh fruit per day could aggravate the condition. Trust your own observations. Notice what helps you feel "clearer" and what causes a coughing, itchy or aggravating response.

BOTANICALS

Echinacea: 30-50 drops up to 6 times a day.

Pau D'Arco	4 parts	For at least 4-6 months,
Quassia	4 parts	use as a combined extract
Licorice	3 parts	20-40 drops, 3-4 times per
Myrrh	3 parts	day.
Yerba Mansa	2 parts	
Black Walnut hulls	2 parts	
Astragalus	1 parts	
Thuja	1 parts	

Garlic: 1 capsule, 3 times per day with meals.

BASIS OF THERAPEUTICS

Echinacea: Increases T-lymphocyte activity. Activates white blood cell response. Increases overall immune system alertness and activity.

Pau D'Arco: Inhibits fungal growth and thus encourages the multiplication of indigenous bacteria.

Quassia: Acts as an antiparasitic agent; stops or prevents growth of other parasites (i.e., giardia, etc.). Also acts as an effective stomach bitter, thereby enhancing digestion.

Licorice: Specifically inhibits the growth of Candida albicans. Decreases inflammation of the respiratory tissues.

Unlike most sweets, it resists fermentation by fungus. Licorice tea is a beverage of choice for any fungus- related problem.

Myrrh: Decreases inflammation of the mucous membranes and bogginess of the lung tissues. Assists Echinacea and Astragalus in their immune system functions.

Yerba Mansa: A mild yet reliable antifungal. Stimulates healing of the mucous tissues of the mouth, digestive tract and lungs. It has an astringent effect on pulmonary connective tissues. Increases fluid transport and utilization in lung tissues.

Black Walnut Hulls: Is one of the best herbal anti-fungals available. It is most effective in the fresh state. It must be taken in small quantities for a minimum of 4-6 months to achieve desired results.

Astragalus: A deep immune system stimulant. Supports the body's effort in controlling the fungus.

Thuja: Like black walnut hulls, this is a very good antifungal agent. The fresh plant must be used.

Garlic: Has antifungal properties. Very specific to Candida albicans. It also has been shown to be effective in treating cryptococcocal meningitis.

SUPPLEMENTS

Caprylic acid (complexed with calcium or magnesium): 1-6 capsules or tablets after meals. Warning: use only with professional guidance especially if there is a history of stomach ulcers or a high cholesterol level.

Acidophilus (Megadophilus): ¼ teaspoon 2-3 times per day at least 1/2 hour before meals.

Biotin: 600 mcg., 1-2 times per day after meals.

Digestive enzymes: 300 mg. after any ample meals.

Zinc: 25-50 mg. once per day after a meal.

Beta-carotene: 10,000 - 30,000 I.U. per day after a meal. See warning note p. 8.

Buffered vitamin C: 500 mg. - 4,000 mg. per day, total, after meals.

Linseed oil (essential fatty acids): 2,500 mgs. per day, after meals.

The following also can be useful in some cases. Magnesium, calcium, selenium, B complex, folic acid, evening primrose oil, iron.

BASIS OF THERAPEUTICS

Caprylic acid: Complexed caprylic acid is a safe, rich source of short chain fatty acids, which specifically discourage fungal growth. It is a potent antifungal agent derived from coconut. When complexed with calcium or magnesium, it primarily releases in the colon, discouraging secondary infection there.

Acidophilus (Megodophilus): Stimulates strong and healthy bacterial colonies in the gut. Prevents the overgrowth of opportunistic fungi, especially Candida albicans.

Biotin: Mechanism poorly understood. Discourages fungal growth.

Digestive enzymes: Promote the complete breakdown of food proteins. This minimizes allergic reactions to half-digested proteins which can leak through a yeast-perforated small intestine. Important in minimizing the secondary food sensitivities seen so often in opportunistic fungal infections.

Zinc: Stimulates the immune system, especially macrophage destruction of fungus in the lungs.

Beta-carotene: Promotes healthy mucous membranes, thereby discouraging the proliferation of fungus. Stimulates lung-mediated immune defenses.

Magnesium: Improves membrane integrity. Magnesium deficiency results in reduced antibody (immune) production.

Calcium: Strengthens cell membranes.

Selenium: Strengthens the immune system. Selenium deficiencies have been found in animals with Candida albicans.

B-Complex: Replaces the nutrients which fungi have been poaching.

Folic acid: Necessary for the formation of white blood cells and lymphocytes, as well as B-cell antibody production. Commonly deficient in Americans.

Essential fatty acids: Stabilize cell membranes. Large amounts are found in the thymus, which initiates T-cell production.

Iron: Stimulates immune response. It can also, in excess, stimulate yeast growth. Therefore it is important to assess the use of iron on an individual basis.

PREVENTION AND HEALING

The rare primary fungal infections can be avoided by taking precautionary steps. Find out if your area harbors a dangerous fungus. People at risk are farmers, archaeologists, earth movers, foundation diggers, and adobe makers. If hazardous fungi are present in your region, wearing a mask when in contact with the soil offers good protection against infection.

Secondary or opportunistic infections can be prevented by eliminating the use of antibiotics, birth control pills, and/or immunosuppressive drugs. Avoid living or working in moldy environments such as old damp houses, greenhouses, bakeries, pizza parlors, or mushroom farms.

Fungi are very slow to grow and also can be very slow to eliminate. Therefore, great patience is required in dealing with a fungal infection. Herbs and supplements may have to be taken for many months to achieve the desired results. Even when all symptoms have disappeared, it is important to keep up the treatment for at least an additional one to two months. This supports the body in totally repairing the damage and in restoring complete health.

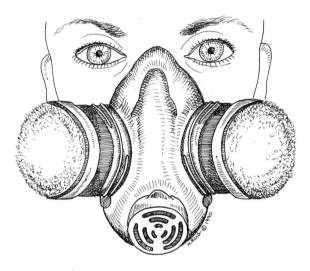

VISUALIZATION

Imagine you are moving through clouds to a bright, light place. The closer you get, the more the clouds lift and dissolve. Now enter this place of brilliance. Breathe in the bright light, allowing it to permeate every cell of your lungs and nasal passages, every cell of your body. The clouds are gone, the brilliance is within you.

AIDS & ARC-RELATED RESPIRATORY INFECTION

If you know or suspect that you have HIV virus, any minor respiratory infection must be taken extremely seriously, even the most benign seeming cough. It is important to act immediately. Create an alive healthy image of yourself and get medical support. The information below is offered as an adjunct to, and not a substitute for, such treatment.

DEFINITION

The most common AIDS related respiratory infection is Pneumocystis carinii pneumonia.

DESCRIPTION

Pneumocystis carinii pneumonia is an acute opportunistic pulmonary infection caused by a protozoan. It occurs in immunosuppressed individuals or in people receiving corticosteroid drugs or immunosuppressive agents. Person-to-person transmission is possible. Malnutrition also is a predisposing factor. Pneumocytosis usually affects only the lungs. It may develop abruptly over two or three days, or its onset may be insidious over several weeks. Difficulty in breathing, chest pain, fever and dry cough are the major symptoms. Untreated, this disease has essentially a 100 percent mortality rate. It must be taken care of promptly.

BIOLOGICAL OVERVIEW

People with HIV virus and a T-cell count below 200 are at high risk for this disease. Minor respiratory symptoms such as shortness of breath, cough and chest pain may develop rapidly into pneumocystis pneumonia. This is avoidable. People at risk should take immediate and effective measures at the onset of ANY respiratory infection, no matter how slight or mild it may seem.

EMOTIONAL INFORMATION

Grief, loss and inertia can initiate a respiratory infection. If you have been experiencing a cycle of grieving and/or a sense of hopelessness, now is the time to confront and move through these feelings with courage.

The profound experience of loss which many survivors of the AIDS/ARC epidemic have had can be complicated by feelings of guilt at having survived. It is important to begin to recognize and release such feelings which "seal in" the grief, making it more difficult to go past it.

Trusting yourself is essential here.

GUIDELINES FOR ACTION

Preventative:

1. Support the immune system.

2. Take care of any infection promptly and thoroughly.

3. Eliminate any debilitating lifestyle factors (see prevention and healing, p. 116).

Treatment:

1. Consult a physician immediately.

2. Rest.

3. Stimulate the immune system.

4. Eliminate the protozoa.

5. Work with the fever (see the COMMON COLD/INFLUENZA, p. 18.)

6. Stabilize and support the lungs.

7. Counterbalance the effects of antibiotics.

THERAPEUTIC RECOMMENDATIONS
FOODS

An alkalizing diet (see the COMMON COLD/INFLUENZA, p. 19) is essential. Alcohol, sugar, coffee, cigarettes, and all drugs, including marijuana, must be eliminated immediately. In most cases eliminating red meat is helpful.

At least five ½ cup servings of fresh vegetables and fruits should be eaten daily. Whether these are taken raw or freshly steamed should be decided by the needs of your constitution, your inclination, and the advice of a trusted health practitioner. Fresh vegetable juices, freshly grated salads, and homemade soups with a vegetable bouillon base are positive choices. Sweet potato is a specific here, as are shitake mushrooms, and carrot juice.

Adequate protein, an average of 40-50 grams per day, is necessary. This can be provided by beans, legumes, seeds, nuts, and small amounts of fresh fish or organic poultry. Dairy foods and eggs are best avoided until you are healed, as they can be congesting to the lungs and lymph glands.

Eat 2 to 5 cloves of raw garlic a day, adding them to as many foods as possible.

If sea vegetables appeal to you, eat them freely up to two (½ cup) servings daily.

For further suggestions, *Healing AIDS Naturally* by L. Badgley, M.D. is useful.

BASIS OF THERAPEUTICS

Alcohol, sugar, coffee, black tea, drugs and red meat are powerfully acidifying. These inhibit the immune system and provide a more hospitable environment for viruses and other microbes. These should be eliminated. Conversely, fresh vegetables and fruits create a supportive and healing alkalizing environment.

Sweet potato is rich in vitamin A and specifically healing to the lungs. Shitake mushrooms contain lentinan, a compound which eliminates HIV virus and antibodies and also has anti-cancer properties. Carrot juice is an excellent source of beta-carotene and potassium.

Low-fat proteins stimulate white blood cells and digestive enzyme production. They also contribute to normal healthy muscle mass.

Raw garlic has an antimicrobial action. It is antiviral, antibacterial, antifungal and antiparasitic. It detoxifies, stimulating cleansing and elimination.

Sea vegetables are a rich source of minerals especially iodine. There is some evidence that iodine may discourage protozoal growth (e.g., iodochlorhydroxyquin, a medically prescribed drug is an antiprotozoal agent).

BOTANICALS

Quassia	4 parts	Take as an extract 40 drops
Pau D'Arco	3 parts	every 3 hours during the
Thuja	2 parts	acute phase.
Garlic	2 parts	

Echinacea	6 parts	Take as an extract up to 60
Osha	4 parts	drops every hour during the
Propolis	3 parts	acute phase.
Ocotillo	2 parts	
Red Root	2 parts	
Spikenard	2 parts	
Poke Root	1 part	
Wild Indigo	1 part	

BASIS OF THERAPEUTICS

Quassia: An anti-protozoic agent. Stimulates the assimilation of nutrients.

Pau D'Arco: Stimulates the immune system to combat infection. Reduces immunosuppression.

Thuja: Decreases protozoan growth and reproduction in affected tissues.

Garlic: A strong antiparasitic agent.

Echinacea: An excellent immune system stimulant. Increases levels of T-4 (a type of white blood cell).

Osha: Supports the respiratory system. Works with the fever, induces perspiration.

Propolis: Prevents or slows down degradation of the tissues under protozan attack.

Ocotillo: A deep immune system stimulant.

Red Root: Stimulates the lymphatic tissues to speed up maturation of the white blood cells.

Spikenard: Increases lymph drainage. Speeds up recuperation of the mucuous membranes of the respiratory system.

Poke Root: Strongly stimulates all aspects of the immune system. Must be taken in small amounts.

Wild Indigo: Best used when the body has difficulty in recovering from an infection. Helps tone up a weary, lethargic defense system.

Preventive: See Immune system tonic, p. 20.

SUPPLEMENTS

Beta-carotene: 25,000 I.U. 1-5 times per day after meals (for a total of 25,000-125,000 I.U. per day) for up to 5 days. EXCEPTION: If you have been taking potent drugs, especially chemical drugs, use a maximum of 50,000 I.U. of beta-carotene to minimize liver toxicity.

Zinc lozenges: 15 mg. 5 times per day for up to two weeks, and 4 times per day thereafter, taken after food. EXCEPTION: If you are anemic (have a low hemoglobin level) use 15 mg., 5 times per day for up to 1 week, then 1 to 2 times per day thereafter.

Buffered Vitamin C: 1,000 - 12,000 mg. per day, up to 500 mg. every ½ hour.

A Good Multiple Vitamin and Mineral Formula: see Appendix D, p. 146.

Garlic: 1 capsule 4 to 6 times per day.

Vitamin E: 800-1200 I.U. per day after a meal. EXCEPTION: If you have high blood pressure, use lesser amounts of vitamin E.

See ABOUT SUPPLEMENTS, p. 8.

Beta-carotene: Supports healthy lung membranes and stimulates antimicrobial action of the immune system's white blood cells. Warning: If the liver is weak from repeated drug use, AZT or hepatitis, high doses, which can overstress the liver critically, should not be taken.

Zinc: Stimulates T-cells and T-helper cells, often inhibited in AIDS and ARC. High doses of zinc (e.g., 75 mg. per day) can compete with iron for absorption and should be used with caution if there is a history of anemia.

Buffered vitamin C: The mechanism of its action is poorly understood. Possibly it enhances interferon, an antiviral compound naturally produced by the immune system. Single doses of 500 mg. of vitamin C are optimally absorbed, saturating the body's pool.

A Good Multiple Vitamin and Mineral Formula: Builds blood and energy. 200 mcg. of selenium, included in such formulas, is vital. Selenium supports the immune system and specifically detoxifies toxins in the lungs related to smoke and air pollution. It also is preventive against a wide variety of cancers and may be useful in preventing Kaposi's sarcoma.

Garlic: See FOODS, p. 114.

Vitamin E: Is anti-inflammatory in the recommended doses. Supports flexibility of the lung tissues and immune strength.

PREVENTION AND HEALING

The aim is to create and/or rebuild a cushion of health around you. In many of people with AIDS or ARC, this cushion has been diminished. While much attention has been focused on the immune system and its functioning or lack thereof, long-term epidemiological evidence suggests that it is the whole body that needs support. Nourishing ourselves effectively and stopping the self-abuses (such as smoking and drinking) which wear away at our cushion of health and confidence are two important steps in self-support.

It is becoming widely recognized that drugs such as alcohol, cocaine, heroin, marijuana, nicotine and amyl nitrate can inhibit the healthy or effective functioning of the immune system and cause specific nutritional deficiencies. Other substances that may look benign— caffeine and sugar, for example—also can cause serious nutritional deficiencies: losses of potassium, chromium, and some of the B vitamins. None of these substances contributes healing energy. At a time when immune strength needs to be maintained or reinforced, clearly they should be eliminated.

Creating your own dietary, exercise and herbal program is vital. This puts you in charge of your own health, and you are the one that needs to be in charge. Many different healing programs are effective. Most include plenty of foods rich in vitamins A and C (see p. 133), high quality low-fat proteins, foods high in fiber and low in fat; moderate exercise (20 minutes, 4 times a week); and herbs similar to those recommended in this section. In this time of blatant and subtle attacks from the media and other sources against people with AIDS/ARC, group support and self-love are important factors in recreating a protective cushion of healing around you.

VISUALIZATION

You are relaxing in a warm, comfortable space. Imagine you are rising to your feet, standing firmly in this place of comfort. As you stand and breathe in and out, freely, regularly, you can begin to imagine a cushion of clear radiant energy forming one-quarter inch from your body, all along your skin. This cushion covers and protects every part of your body, especially your lungs, spine, heart, and pelvis. As you breathe in and out, you can imagine that this cushion grows, becoming wider, softer, more vibrant. Allow it to grow to one-half inch, an inch, two inches or more. If you like, you can imagine this cushion of healing extending two to three feet beyond the boundaries of your body. Relax in this cushion as much as you like, and wear it as often as you please.

HIV: Human Immunodeficiency Virus; one of the viruses found in many ARC and AIDS patients.

ARC: AIDS Related Complex; a group of symptoms which is found in some people who test HIV positive.

AIDS: Acquired Immune Deficiency Syndrome; an illness in which the body becomes infected with different germs as the result of weakened body resistance.

SMOKING: HOW TO STOP

DEFINITION

"To draw in and exhale smoke from a cigarette, cigar, pipe, or the like." The American Heritage Dictionary

DESCRIPTION

Most of the ills caused by smoking are familiar to smokers and non-smokers alike. Packages of cigarettes are littered with warnings and most public places now prohibit smoking. During the last ten years, strong pressure has been exerted on smokers to quit their habit and these social and economic pressures are likely to intensify. This section is designed to support the smoker in his/her own choice to stop smoking.

BIOLOGICAL OVERVIEW

Smoking has a powerful impact not only on the lungs, but on the functioning of the whole body. Therefore any program to break this habit should address all of the affected areas.

Each time something is taken into the mouth—and this includes cigarettes—the whole gastro-intestinal tract is stimulated. Digestive secretions increase and intestinal transit time is shortened. When smoking is stopped, this stimulation stops. There is a decrease in digestive juices, often resulting in constipation. Some people begin to eat candy or food in compensation for the lost oral stimulation of smoking. Weight gain is possible and usually preventable in these circumstances.

Before smokers start the smoking habit, they tend to have higher EEG levels (brain activity) and higher levels of the circulating adrenal catecholamines, epinephrine and norepinephrine. They tend to be more high-strung than non-smokers. Nicotine acts as a sedative, a buffer between the smoker's rapid thought processes and the intensity of environmental stimuli. A stop-smoking program must take this factor into consideration. Calming herbs and supplements are recommended.

Tobacco smoke acts as a cilia stimulant, and stimulates the production of a thicker, more viscous protective mucus. There is increased lubrication of the pleura by serous fluids. In a long-term smoker, smoke also acts as a bronchial dilator. When smoking is stopped, this artificial stimulation/ irritation is lost. Therefore, it is important to take herbal pulmonary stimulants at this time. The lungs are usually in a depressed state for a period of two weeks to a month after the cessation of smoking.

Smoking also stimulates the release of glucose into the blood stream. Withdrawal from the habit often initially induces symptoms of hypoglycemia. Appropriate foods can minimize these temporary symptoms.

It is the liver's role to detoxify the circulating nicotine into harmless compounds. Stimulating this organ helps to decrease the nicotine craving that accompanies withdrawal.

EMOTIONAL INFORMATION

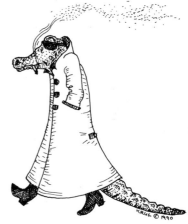

Smokers often reach for a cigarette when they are tense. This is understandable since smoking has a sedative effect. However, cigarettes do not process feelings; they simply help to relax you when feelings of anger, sadness or loving that you choose not to face arise. So, as you quit, many unprocessed feelings which may have been stored for decades can begin to emerge. You may find yourself more irritable, edgy, vulnerable, or at a loss to know how you feel. While some of this is a biological reaction to nicotine withdrawal, it also has to do with the release of long-repressed feelings, many of them uncomfortable.

Facing and coming to terms with these feelings is not an instant process. Many ex-smokers find themselves facing unexpected emotions six months or more after they have quit. It is important to understand that this generally is part of the extended withdrawal process and that it is important to your healing and cleansing.

As the difficult emotions surface, it can be especially easy to start smoking again. You've kicked the habit physically, but the emotional work is still before you. After all the effort of freeing yourself physically, this emotional challenge can sometimes feel like more than you can handle. Now is the time to create support for yourself: exercise to help the feelings move out, seek counseling or group support. Find whatever feels most appropriate for you, but get the help you need. The emotional maturation you will experience is well worth the effort.

Often ex-smokers look back in amazement at the emotional habits into which they had locked themselves in the time when they smoked. They now see the unnecessary restrictions they had placed on themselves, masking their true feelings with the false "feel-goodness" of smoke.

As we see it, quitting smoking is an initiation process. To physically stop smoking is to conquer the first "dragon at the gate." The second dragon at the threshold is the emotional work to be done. Facing and moving past this great challenge richly repays your effort.

GUIDELINES FOR ACTION

1. Stop smoking.

2. Avoid the circumstances, times, and conditions which promote smoking (see prevention and healing p. 125.)

3. Stimulate the elimination of nicotine from the body by:
   a) drinking plenty of fluids;
   b) taking 1-2 walks in fresh air daily, for at least 15 minutes each time;
   c) using the foods, herbs and supplements suggested in

therapeutic recommendations below.

4. Satisfy oral stimulation needs in a healing way.

5. Stimulate the digestive system and prevent constipation.

6. Calm and support the nervous system.

7. Stimulate the respiratory system.

8. Get group support.

THERAPEUTIC RECOMMENDATIONS
FOODS

It is important to choose foods that are texturally, physically and emotionally appealing yet relatively low in fat content. Fat slows down the digestive processes, which already have been slowed by withdrawal from smoking. Fresh fruits are high in fiber, often rich in vitamins A and C, and provide the needed fluids to flush excess nicotine from the system. Figs and prunes can be especially useful. Fruit juices, diluted one-to-one with water to cut their sweetness, also are helpful.

Onion dip made with one tablespoon of plain, low-fat yogurt and one cup of ricotta cheese per packet of dip provides a calming and nutritious way to eat crunchy vegetables or high-fiber crackers. Review the foods rich in vitamins A, B and C (see Appendix C, p. 133) and choose those most satisfying to you. Oat bran muffins, carrot juice and sunflower seeds are particularly helpful snacks.

BASIS OF THERAPEUTICS

Low-fat, high fiber foods, particularly figs and prunes, stimulate peristalsis and thereby promote digestion and elimination. High fiber foods like oat bran muffins, whole grain crackers, fresh fruit and vegetables and sunflower seeds also can help reduce cholesterol levels, which are often elevated in smokers. Carrot and fruit juices provide the extra vitamin A and C that ex-smokers need. Ricotta cheese and yogurt are rich sources of calcium, which calm the nerves. These low-fat foods also provide protein to alleviate the temporary hypoglycemia which can arise after stopping smoking.

BOTANICALS

Lobelia	6 parts	Take as a combined extract 20-30 drops every 2-4 hours during the first 4 weeks.
Oats	4 parts	
Osha	4 parts	
Pleurisy Root	2 parts	
Grindelia	1 parts	
Mullein	1 part	

Licorice Root, sliced: one slice as often as needed. Slowly suck on the root for oral stimulation.

Psyllium husk powder: 1 teaspoonful in a full glass of water once or twice a day.

Gentian root: 10 drops 20 minutes before meals.

Passion flower: 20-40 drops not more often than every 2 hours, as needed.

Woodsgrown American Ginseng: 20 drops, 3 times a day.

BASIS OF THERAPEUTICS

Lobelia: Contains lobeline, a powerful respiratory stimulant. Lobeline also stimulates the same receptor sites as nicotine. Extremely helpful in alleviating withdrawal symptoms.

Oats: Excellent nervous system tonic. Calms withdrawal symptoms.

Osha: Acts as a bronchial dilator. Stimulates the cilia's removal of mucus from the lungs.

Pleurisy Root: Stimulates proper mucus production and lubrication of the pleura by serous fluids.

Grindelia: Liquifies mucus and facilitates its expectoration.

Mullein: Relieves bronchial irritation and cough.

Licorice Root: Satisfies the need for oral stimulation. It also offers adrenal support and helps to stabilize the blood sugar level. Mildly laxative.

Psyllium husk powder: Helps prevent constipation. Normalizes intestinal transit time. It is an intestinal bulk forming agent.

Gentian: As a bitter tonic, it stimulates gastric juice production.

Passion flower: Calms nervous tension and facilitates sleep. Provides a cushion in cases of excessive stimulation.

Woodsgrown American Ginseng: Induces a feeling of well-being. Supports the adrenal glands. Normalizes blood sugar levels by stimulating pancreatic release of glucogen.

SUPPLEMENTS

L-cysteine: 500 mg., two to three times per day before meals.

A Good Multiple Vitamin and Mineral Formula: See Appendix D, p. 146.

Buffered vitamin C: 1,000-3,000 mg. per day taken after meals.

Beta-carotene: 10,000-25,000 I.U. per day after a meal.

Selenium: 200 mcg. once per day after a meal.

Zinc: 50 mg. once per day after a meal.

BASIS OF THERAPEUTICS

L-cysteine: Like Grindelia, liquifies mucus and facilitates its expectoration. May assist in reversing some types of cross-linkage of tissue, thereby easing "smoker's wrinkles."

A Good Multiple Vitamin and Mineral Formula: Is used here especially for its high B complex content. Niacin promotes blood vessel dilation and reduces cholesterol, thereby addressing two problems common to smokers: constricted blood vessels and elevated cholesterol. Vitamin B_6 levels are lower in smokers than in non-smokers. Pantothenic acid helps clear congested sinus tissues.

Buffered vitamin C: Speeds excretion of nicotine and provides needed antioxidant support for the respiratory system. Can promote elimination.

Beta-carotene: Is deficient in smokers. This deficiency is viewed as one possible underlying cause for the increased rate of lung cancer in smokers. Supports and heals mucous membranes.

Selenium: A potent cancer preventive. Detoxifies heavy metals commonly found in tobacco.

Zinc: Prevents infection. Promotes ability to taste.

ADDITIONAL SUPPORT

Air filters remove past and present tobacco odors from the environment. Such odors can be irritating and also can trigger nicotine cravings.

PREVENTION AND HEALING

Humans are creatures of habit. Most cigarettes are smoked without the smoker being fully aware of the action. One way to stop smoking is to become conscious of the process every time you light a cigarette and smoke it, taking the time to see what is happening emotionally and physically.

Still another suggestion is to alter your way of doing things you associate with smoking. If after a meal you usually have a cup of coffee and a cigarette, get up instead and go for a short walk. If you stay at the table, it will be harder to resist that after-meal cigarette. By changing the habitual actions around it, the smoking habit is thrown off balance and becomes easier to break.

When the desire for a cigarette comes on, deep breathing and vigorous exercise are extremely helpful. Brisk walks in fresh air, taking deep breaths as you go, will dilate the bronchioles, relax the nerves, change the focus, and positively alter the body's energy patterns.

Support groups also can help you in your undertaking. They offer a safe space in which to share the feelings that surface.

Know that for up to a year you may feel challenged in your decision to stop smoking. Be gentle and patient with yourself and your tensions during this process. Yet also know that you must be rock solid in holding to your commitment to yourself. Once you have quit, you will find that environments that are calming to you will play an important role in reinforcing your decision.

Breaking Free of Compulsive Eating by Geneen Roth is a useful secondary support if oral cravings begin to feel overwhelming.

VISUALIZATION

You are breathing in and out. Fully expand and relax your chest as you breathe. Imagine yourself as you were when you were a small child, before you ever smoked. Imagine this child is in your heart now as you breathe. Send this small precious self love and energy, clean fresh air. Then imagine that the adult self has joined the child self in your heart. Send loving to every part of you as you breathe.

NOTES

APPENDIX A
BREATHING EXERCISES

The purpose of these breathing exercises is threefold:

1) Increase the amount of oxygen that will reach the alveolar tissues and increase the amount of oxygen excreted from the lungs.

2) Increase the efficiency and strength of the diaphragm.

3) Re-educate yourself into a well-coordinated and efficient breathing pattern to decrease the effort of breathing.

In a healthy person, the diaphragm is responsible for 65 to 70% of respiration while the chest and accessory respiratory muscles only account for 30 to 35%. In the person with Chronic Obstructive Pulmonary Disease the lungs lose their elasticity and their recoiling properties and become distended. The diaphragm also becomes weakened and depressed. This condition, when left on its destructive course will progress until the chest and accessory muscles carry 70% of the respiratory effort and the diaphragm only 30%. The following exercises will increase your breathing capacity substantially.

ABDOMINAL BREATHING

Lie on your back with your legs bent. Place one hand on your chest. The other hand goes on your abdomen; your thumb should be just slightly lower than your navel (belly button). Now breathe deeply through your nose. Feel your abdomen rise fully under your bottom hand. Your chest should remain stationary, not expanded. Exhale slowly through pursed lips, your abdomen will fall to the floor, assisted by the pressure of your bottom hand. Do this exercise three minutes morning and evening until you master it without the help of your hands.

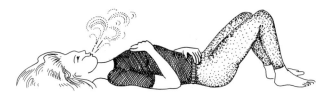

• BASIC ABDOMINAL BREATHING

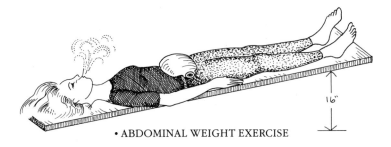

• ABDOMINAL WEIGHT EXERCISE

You can also repeat this exercise lying on each side with your legs drawn up. Do this for up to three minutes each side.

A metronome may be used to time your breathing.

1½ seconds to breath in

3 seconds to breath out

Abdominal Weight Exercise

Raise the foot of a bed about 16 inches. Place a 1 pound weight (preferably a bag of sand, earth or marbles, not books or water bottle) on your abdomen. Do the basic abdominal breathing, this time pushing the abdomen against the weight as you exhale. Do this exercise for 5 to 10 minutes twice a day. Every fourth day add ½ pound of weight until the bag reaches 5 pounds.

Lower Rib Expansion and Constriction

Place a strip of cloth about 5 feet long around your lower ribs, ends crossed. Do the basic abdominal breathing exercise. Let the belt out when you breathe in.

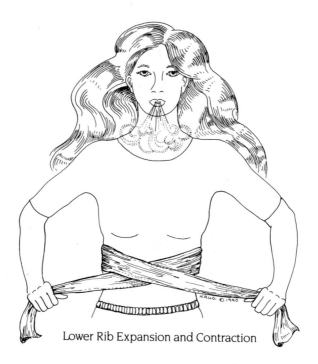

Lower Rib Expansion and Contraction

Tighten it firmly (not excessively) as you breathe out. First, do this exercise sitting down, then do it standing and finally while walking around the room. When walking take one step with inhalation and two steps with expiration. Practice until you can do these chest movements without the belt and without thinking about it.

Candle Blowing

This exercise is first done in a sitting position. Position a lighted candle on the table so that the flame is at the height of the mouth and about 5 inches away. Blow gently through pursed lips. Keep your chest stationary while you exhale, drawing your abdomen inward. Do not extinguish the flame but simply bend it away from you. Try to maintain a steady bent flame. Do this for three minutes at bedtime. Increase distance three inches nightly until you

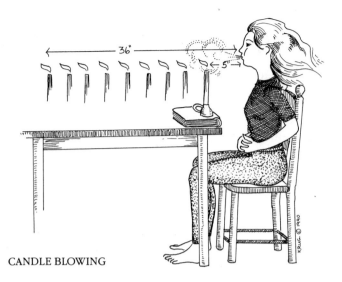

CANDLE BLOWING

are able to be three feet away from the candle. Once this is mastered (after one month or more), start again, this time standing. Bring flame to mouth level. Repeat exercise.

APPENDIX B
AMADEA'S HEALING BROTH

1½ c. fresh vegetables: carrots, broccoli, dark leafy greens and/or parsley
2 stalks celery
1/4 c. raw sunflower seeds
1 heaping tsp. mellow white or yellow miso
2½ c. water

Place water and steamer in pot and bring water to a boil. Place vegetables in the steamer. Cover. Steam 5-8 minutes until their color is vivid, not drab (the latter is an indicator of overdoneness). While steaming the vegetables, grind dry sunflower seeds to a powder in blender. Add the steamed vegetables, cooking water, and miso and blend on medium for 30 seconds.

This high-zinc formula replenishes vitamins A and C, as well as potassium and magnesium electrolytes. It is specifically designed to be non-mucus forming, and is soothing to the gut and mucosa.

APPENDIX C
FOODS HIGH IN NUTRIENTS

VITAMIN A

Food	CALMS VPK	Amount	Preparation	Amount of Nutrient
Apricots	VK	3 med.	raw	2,890 IU
Beef liver, organic	V	¼ lb.		11,000
Beet greens	K	1 cup	cooked	7,400
Broccoli	PK	1 cup	cooked	3,800
Butter, salted	V			
unsalted	P			
grazing		¼ lb.		5,000
hay in winter		¼ lb.		1,000
Cantaloupe	VP	¼ med.	raw	3,400
Carrot	VK	1 med.	raw	10,000
juice		1 cup		24,750
Chard	K	1 cup	cooked	7,830
Chicken liver, organic	V	¼ lb.		13,825
Chili powder	VK	1 tsp.		900
red	VK	½ cup	canned	11,750
Cod-liver oil		1 tbsp.		11,900
Crab		¼ lb.	steamed	2,450
Dandelion greens	PK	1 cup	cooked	10,400
Kale	PK	1 cup	cooked	9,130
Lamb's liver, organic	V	¼ lb.		57,270
Lamb's quarters	K	1 cup	cooked	19,000
Lettuce				
leaf		¼ head	raw	1,900
romaine	PK	4 leaves	raw	1,400
iceberg (for comparison)		¼ head		300
Mango	VPK	1 med.		11,090
Mustard greens	K	1 cup	cooked	14,760
Nori	V	3½ oz.		11,000
Papaya	V	½ med.	raw	2,625
Paprika	VK	1 tsp.		1,270
Parsley	VPK	1 oz.		1,830
Persimmon	K	1 med.	raw	4,600
Pumpkin	V	1 cup	canned	15,860
Spinach	K	1 cup	cooked	14,580
Squash,				
butternut	VP	1 cup	baked	13,000

hubbard	VP	1 cup	baked	9,800
Sweet potato	VP	1 aver.	baked	9,230
Turnip greens	K	1 cup	cooked	9,140
Watermelon	P	slice 1x6½"	raw	3,540

VITAMIN B COMPLEX
(These foods are rich sources of vitamin B complex.)
Brewer's yeast
Chicken
Egg yolk
Fruits (fresh, raw)
Legumes
Milk
Organ meats (heart, liver, kidneys)
Peanuts
Soybeans
Wheat germ
Whey
Whole grains

VITAMIN B$_6$ (PYRIDOXINE)

Food	CALMS VPK	Amount	Preparation	Amount of Nutrient
Avocado	VP	½ med.	fresh	.46
Bananas	V	3½ oz.	fresh	.51
Beans				
garbanzo	PK	½ cup	dry	.54
lima	PK	½ cup	dry	.52
navy	PK	½ cup	dry	.57
Beef				
ground, lean		¼ lb.		.50 mg.
kidney		¼ lb.		1.00
liver		¼ lb.		1.00
Blueberries	VPK	1 cup	fresh	1.00
Brazil nuts	V	1 cup	raw	.29
Buckwheat flour	K	1 cup	dark	.58
Chestnuts		1 cup	fresh	.53
Chicken breast	VP	¼ lb.		.77
Corn	PK	1 cup	cooked	.47
Halibut	V	¼ lb.		.50
Hazelnuts	V	1 cup	raw	.74
Kale	PK	½ lb.	fresh	.68

Lentils	P	½ cup	dry	.57
Mackerel	V	¼ lb.		.75
Orange juice	V	1 cup	fresh	1.00
Peanuts		1 cup	roasted	.58
Rice bran	VPK	⅓ cup		.80
Rice, brown	V	1 cup	raw	1.00
Rice polishings		¼ cup		.80
Salmon		¼ lb.		.79
Soybeans	P	3½ oz.	raw	.81
Soy flour	P	1 cup	defatted	1.00
Spinach	K	½ lb.	fresh	.64
Sunflower seeds	VPK	1 cup		1.80
Tomato juice		1 cup		.37
Trout	V	¼ lb.		.78
Tuna	V	3/12 oz.	canned	.43
Walnuts	V	3½ oz.		.73
Wheat germ	V	1 cup	toasted	1.10
Yeast, torula		1 oz.		.84

FOLIC ACID

Food	CALMS VPK	Amount	Preparation	Amount of Nutrient
Asparagus	VPK	5-6 spears		.64 mg
Avocado	VP	½ med.		.41
Beets	VK	2 med.		.93
Brussels sprouts	PK	3 large		.97
Brewer's yeast		1 tbsp.		.19
Bulgur	VP	¼ cup	dry	7.70
Cantaloupe	VP	1 cup	diced	.49
Chicken liver, organic	V	¼ lb.		.41
Fenugreek seeds	VK	1 tsp.		2.11
Garbanzo beans	PK	1 cup	raw	.40
Grapefruit juice	V	1 cup		.52
Lettuce, romaine	PK	1 cup	cut	1.02
Orange juice	V	1 cup	fresh	1.64
Rye	K	1 cup	dark	.99
Soybeans	P	½ cup	dry	2.36
Soy flour	P	1 cup	full-fat	.31
Spinach	K	½ lb.		4.63
Sweet potato	VP	1 med.		.84
Wheat germ		1 cup	raw	.33
		1 cup	toasted	.42

Wheat, whole	VP	1 cup	stirred	.80
Yeast				
active dry		1 tbsp.		2.86
brewer's		1 tbsp.		3.08

PANTOTHENIC ACID

Food	CALMS VPK	Amount	Preparation	Amount of Nutrient
Anchovies		3	fillets	2.32 mg
Asparagus	VPK	1 cup	raw	.84
Avocado	VP	1 aver.	raw	2.10
Beef				
brain, organic		¼ lb.		2.90
heart, organic		¼ lb.		2.80
kidney, organic		¼ lb.		4.40
liver, organic	¼ lb.		8.70	
Broccoli	PK	1 piece	raw	1.20
Buckwheat flour	K	3½ oz.	dark	1.45
Cabbage	PK	1 cup	raw	1.10
Cashews	V	1 cup	roasted	1.82
Cheese, cottage	VP	1 cup	2% fat	.55
Chicken liver, organic	V	¼ lb.		6.80
Chili, red	VK	½ cup	canned	1.30
Eggs	V	1 large		.99
Flounder	V	¼ lb.		.98
Hazelnuts	V	1 cup	roasted	1.82
Herring	V	¼ lb.	fresh	1.40
Lentils	P	½ cup	dry	1.30
Lobster		¼ lb.		1.50
Milk, skim	VP	1 cup		.81
Peanuts		3½ oz.	raw	2.80
Peas		3½ oz.	dry	2.00
Pecans		1 cup	roasted	1.82
Rice polishings	VPK	¼ cup		1.60
Salmon		¼ lb.	fresh	1.40
Soybeans	P	3½ oz.	dry, raw	1.70
Soy flour	P	1 cup	defatted	3.06
Sunflower seeds	VPK	1 cup		2.00
Trout, rainbow	V	¼ lb.		2.20
Wheat bran	P	3½ oz.	100%	2.90
Yeast, brewer's		1 tbsp.		1.20

| Yeast, torula | | 1 oz. | | 3.10 |
| Yogurt | V | 8 oz. | skim, plain | 1.34 |

VITAMIN C

Food	CALMS VPK	Amount	Preparation	Amount of Nutrient
Asparagus	VPK	⅔ cup	cooked	26 mg
Bell pepper, green	PK	1 large	fresh	128
red		1 med.	fresh	150
Blackberries	VPK	½ cup	fresh	15
Broccoli	PK	⅔ cup	cooked	90
Brussels sprouts	PK	6-8 med.	cooked	87
Cabbage	PK	⅗ cup	cooked	33
Cantaloupe	VP	½ melon		90
Cauliflower	PK	⅞ cup	cooked	55
Chili, red	VK	3 ½ oz.	fresh	369
Collard greens		1 cup	cooked	140
Dandelion greens	PK	3 ½ oz.	fresh	35
Guava		1 med.	fresh	165
Honeydew melon	VP	¼ small	fresh	23
Kale	PK	¾ cup	cooked	62
Kiwi	V	1 med.	fresh	75
Lemon	V	1 med.	fresh	31
Mango	VPK	1 med.	fresh	57
Orange				
navel	V	1 med.	fresh	80
(P if sweet)				
valencia		1 med.	fresh	59
Orange juice	V	8 oz.	fresh	124
		8 oz.	frozen	97
Papaya	V	1 med.	fresh	188
Parsley	VPK	1 tbsp.	fresh, chopped	17
Pineapple	V	1 cup	fresh	24
Potato	PK	1 large	baked	30
Raspberries	VK	1 cup	fresh	31
Sorrel	K	½ cup	cooked	54
Spinach	K	1 cup	cooked	50
Strawberries	VK	1 cup	fresh	85
Sweet Potato	VP	1 large	baked	40
Tomato		1 med.	fresh	34

BIOFLAVONOIDS
Rich Sources:
Apricots (VK)
Bell peppers (with white core) (PK)
Blackberries (VPK)
Black currants
Broccoli (PK)
Buckwheat (K)
Cantaloupe (VP)
Cherries (VK, P if sweet)
Citrus fruits (skins and pulps)
Grapes (V, P if sweet)
Onions, red (K, V if cooked)
Papaya (V)
Parsley (VPK)
Plums (V, P if sweet)
Prunes (PK)
Rose hips
Tomatoes
Walnuts

VITAMIN E

Food	CALMS VPK	Amount	Preparation	Amount of Nutrient
Almonds	V	¼ cup		13 IU
Asparagus	VPK	5-6 spears		4
Beet greens	K	½ lb.		7
Blackberries, wild	VPK	1 cup		9
Hazelnuts	V	¼ cup		12
Kale	PK	3 ½ oz.	fresh	8
Leeks	VK	3-4		5
Lobster		3 oz.		2
Peanut Butter		2 tbsp.		4
Peanuts		1 cup	toasted, w/skins	13
Pecans	V	¼ cup		13
Safflower oil		1 tbsp.		8
Salmon	V	3 oz.		2
Spinach	K	½ lb.		11
Sunflower oil	VP	1 tbsp.		13
Sunflower seeds	VPK	¼ cup		27
Tuna, light	V	6½ oz.	canned in oil	5

Turnip greens	K	½ lb.		8
Walnut oil	V	1 tbsp.		13
Wheat germ	V	½ cup	fresh	13
Wheat germ oil	V	1 tbsp.		40

ESSENTIAL FATTY ACIDS

Food	CALMS VPK	Amount	Preparation	Linoleic Acid Content (Omega-6)
Black walnuts	V	100 gms.		28 gms.
Corn oil	VK	100 gms.		53 gms.
English walnuts	V	100 gms.		40 gms.
Peanut oil		100 gms.		29 gms.
Safflower oil	V	100 gms.		72 gms.
Sesame seeds	V	100 gms.		22 gms.
Soybean oil	VP	100 gms.		52 gms.
Sunflower seeds	VPK	100 gms.		30 gms.

				Linolenic Acid Content (Omega-3)
Cod-liver oil	V	100 gms.		19 gms.
Eel, American	V	¼ lb.		8 gms.
Mackerel, Atlantic	V	¼ lb.		10 gms.
Purslane	VPK	100 gms.		9 gms.
Salmon				
Chinook	V	¼ lb.	canned	13 gms.
Pink	V	¼ lb.		9 gms.

L-CYSTEINE

Rich Sources:

Alfalfa	Garlic
Apples	Hazelnuts
Beets	Horseradish
Brazilnuts	Kale
Brussels sprouts	Onion
Cabbage	Pineapple
Carrot	Raspberry
Cauliflower	
Currants	
Filberts	

CALCIUM

Food	CALMS VPK	Amount	Preparation	Amount of Nutrient
Almonds	V	1 cup	raw	332 mg
Beans, black	PK	1 cup	dry	270
Beet greens	K	3½ oz.	cooked	99
Broccoli	PK	1 med. stalk	cooked	158
Buttermilk	V	1 cup		300
Cheese				
cottage	VP	1 cup		230
ricotta	VP	1 cup	part skim	669
Swiss	V	2 oz.		544
Collards	PK	3½ oz.	cooked	152
Dandelion greens	PK	½ cup	fresh	180
		½ cup	cooked	147
Dulse	V	3½ oz.		567
Garbanzo beans	PK	1 cup	dry	300
Hazelnuts	V	1 cup	raw	282
Hijiki	V	3½ oz.		1400
Kale	PK	½ cup	cooked	103
Kombu	V	3½ oz.		800
Milk				
cow	VP	1 cup	whole	291
cow	VP	1 cup	skim	302
goat	PK	1 cup		326
human	VPK	1 cup		80
Miso	V	3½ oz.		308
Molasses, blackstrap	V	1 tbsp.		137
Salmon, sockeye	V	3 oz.	drained solids	274
Scallops	V	¼ lb.	frozen	449
Sesame seeds	V	½ cup		580
Shrimp	V	¼ lb.	fresh	249
Tofu	VP	3 oz.		109
Turnip greens	K	3½ oz.	cooked	184
Wakame	V	3½₁ oz.		1300
Yogurt	VK	1 cup		452

IRON

Food	CALMS VPK	Amount	Preparation	Amount of Nutrient
Beans,				
black	PK	⅓ cup	cooked	5.2
garbanzo	PK	1 cup	cooked	6.9
pinto	PK	⅓ cup	cooked	4.1
Beef, lean, organic		¼ lb.	ground	13.0
Chicken liver, organic	V	¼ lb.		9.5
Coconut milk	VP	1 cup		3.8
Cumin	VPK	1 tsp.		1.4
Dandelion greens	PK	3 ½ oz.	fresh	3.1
Dulse		3 ½ oz.		6.3
Fenugreek	VK	1 tsp.		1.2
Hijiki	V	3 ½ oz.		29.0
Jerusalem artichokes	PK	3 ½ oz.		3.4
Kombu	V	3 ½ oz.		10.0
Lettuce				
butterhead	PK	3 ½ oz.	raw	2.0
Millet	K	1 cup		15.5
Miso	V	3 ½ oz.		60.0
Molasses,				
blackstrap	V	1 tbsp.		3.2
Nori	V	3 ½ oz.	12.0	
Oysters		¼ lb.	fresh	6.1
Peas, split	PK	1 cup	dry	10.2
Persimmons,				
native	K	3 ½ oz.		2.5
Potato flour	K	1 cup		18.9
Prune juice	PK	1 cup		10.5
Pumpkin seeds	V	¼ cup		4.4
(P & K in mod.)				
Rice bran	VPK	¼ cup		4.8
Sesame seeds	V	½ cup		5.2
Soy flour	P	1 cup	defatted	15.3
Spinach	K	3 ½ oz.	fresh	3.1
	K	3 ½ oz.	cooked	2.2
Thyme	VK	1 tsp.		1.7
Tomato juice		1 cup		2.2
Venison	V	¼ lb.		5.7
Wheat bran	P	¼ cup	raw	2.2

MAGNESIUM

Food	CALMS VPK	Amount	Preparation	Amount of Nutrient
Almonds	V	¼ cup		96 mg
Avocado	VP	½ med.		56
Banana	V	1 med.		58
Barley	PK	3 ½ oz.	whole grain	124
Beans				
kidney	P	¼ cup	dried, cooked	82
soy	P	¼ cup	dried	138
Beet greens	K	3 ½ oz.	fresh	106
Brazil nuts	V	3 ½ oz.		225
Buckwheat	K	3 ½ oz.		229
Cashews	V	¼ cup		94
Chard, Swiss	K	½ lb.		148
Chocolate		1 oz.	bitter or baking	82
Dandelion greens	PK	½ lb.		82
Molasses, blackstrap	V	1 tbsp.		52
Oatmeal	VP	1 cup		50
Peanut butter		2 tbsp.		56
Peppers				
chili, red	VK	¼ cup	canned	104
chili, green	VK	¼ cup	canned	7
green	PK	3 ½ oz.	fresh	169
Potato	PK	1 med.		51
Prunes	PK	1 cup	cooked, unsweetened	50
Sesame seeds	V	3 ½ oz.	fresh, whole	181
Shrimp		4 oz.		48
Snails		3 ½ oz.		250
Sole		4 oz.		34
Soy flour		½ cup		155
Spinach	K	½ cup	cooked, drained	56
		½ cup	fresh	22
Tofu	VP	3 oz.		95
Walnuts, black		3 ½ oz.		190

Watermelon	P	slice	6x1 ½"	48
Wheat bran	P	¼ cup	fresh	69
germ		¼ cup	fresh	84
whole flour	VP	½ cup		68

SELENIUM

Food	CALMS VPK	Amount	Preparation	Amount of Nutrient
Barley, pearled	PK	3 ½ oz.		38 mcg.
Beef				
kidney, organic		¼ lb.		160
liver, organic		¼ lb.		51
Black-eyed peas	PK	½ cup	canned	24
Brazil nuts	V	1 cup	fresh	144
Bread				
whole wheat	V	1 slice		16
Cashews	V	3 ½ oz.		68
Chicken liver, organic	V	3 ½ oz.		71
Cod		¼ lb.		47
Egg	V	1 med.	fresh	12
Flounder	V	¼ lb.		38
Lobster		¼ lb.		118
Molasses	V	3 ½ oz.		128
Mushrooms	PK	1 cup	canned, drained	29
Oysters		¼ lb.	fresh	55
Peanuts		3 ½ oz.	roasted	38
		3 ½ oz.	fresh	3
Potato Chips, bacon & sour cream, Ruffles brand		1 oz.		386
Just couldn't resist!				
Rice, brown	V	1 cup	fresh	77
Scallops	V	¼ lb.		87
Shrimp	V	¼ lb.	fresh	227
Tuna	V	3 ½ oz.	canned	115
Wheat bran	PK	1 cup	fresh	36
flour	VP	1 cup	all purpose	22
germ	V	1 cup	fresh	83

ZINC

Food	CALMS VPK	Amount	Preparation	Amount of Nutrient
Beef				
lean, organic		3 oz.		5.3 mg.
liver, organic		3 oz.		4.4
Cheese, Swiss	V	2 oz.		2.2
Chicken hearts, organic	V	3 oz.		6.3
Herring	V	3½ oz.		70.0-120.0
Kelp	V	1 tbsp.	powdered	2.4
Lobster		3½ oz.		7.9
Maple syrup	VP	3½ oz.		5.2-10.5
Milk, dry,				
nonfat		1 cup		3.1
Oatmeal	VP	3½ oz.		14.0
Oysters		3½ oz.		160.0
Peanuts		3½ oz.		3.2
Peas	PK	3½ oz.		3.5
Pumpkin seeds	V	¼ cup		2.6
(P&K in mod.)				
Rice bran	VPK	1 cup		3.1
Wheat bran	P	3½ oz.		14.0
germ	V	¼ cup	toasted	3.2

REFERENCES

Understanding Vitamins and Minerals, by the Editors of *Prevention Magazine*, Rodale Press, Emmaus, PA, 1984

Henderson, Sybil, *Quick and Easy Nutritional Guide for Fresh Fruits and Vegetables*, Henderson Publications, Los Angeles, CA, 1971

Nutrition Almanac, Nutrition Search, Inc., McGraw-Hill, 1979

Kroeger, Hanna, *Instant Herbal Locator*, 1979

Pennington, Jean A.T. and Church, Helen Nichols, *Bowes and Churche's Food Values of Portions Commonly Used*, Fourteenth Edition, J. B. Lippincott Cot, Philadelphia, 1985

Kroeger, Hanna, *Instant Vitamin-Mineral Locator*, 1972

Heritage, Ford, *Composition and Facts about Foods*, republished by Health Research, Mokelumne Hill, CA, 1971

Watt, Bernia K. and Merrill, Annabel L., *Handbook of the Nutritional Contents of Foods*, for U. S. Dept of Agriculture, Dover Publ, Inc., NY, original 1963; reprint 1975

Tver, David F. and Russell, Percy, *The Nutrition and Health Encyclopedia*, Van Nostrand Reinhold Co., NY, 1981

Kutsky, Roman, *Handbook of Vitamins, Minerals and Hormones*, Second Edition, Van Nostrand Reinhold Co., NY, 1981

Rodale, J. I. and Staff, *The Complete Book of Food and Nutrition*, Rodale Books, Inc., Emmaus, PA, 1971

The Complete Book of Vitamins, by the Staff of Prevention Magazine, Rodale Press, Emmaus, PA, 1977

Robertson, Laurel, Flinders, Carol and Godfrey, Bronwen, *Laurel's Kitchen*, Bantam Books, Inc., NY, 1978

Krause, Marie and Mahan, Kathleen, *Food, Nutrition and Diet Therapy*, 7th Ed., W. B. Saunders Co., 1984

Journal of the American Dietetic Association

☆VPK

Refers to a healing system practiced in India. This system called Ayurveda comprises three basic types of biological energies which determine individual constitution, Vata, Pita and Kapha. For more information consult *The Ayurvedic Cookbook* by Amadea Morningstar.

APPENDIX D
A GOOD MULTIPLE VITAMIN AND MINERAL FORMULA

NUTRIENTS	CHILDREN (2-12)	ADULTS
Beta-carotene (Vitamin A activity)	4,000 I.U.	10,000 I.U.
Vitamin D	200-400 I.U.	100-400 I.U.
Vitamin E	30-150 I.U.	200-600 I.U.
Vitamin C	50-500 mg.	250-1,000 mg.
Vitamin B-1	5-25 mg.	25-75 mg.
Vitamin B-2	3-13 mg.	15-50 mg.
Niacin (and/or niacinamide)	10-50 mg.	50-150 mg.
Pantothenic acid	20-150 mg.	50-500 mg.
Vitamin B-6	3-12 mg.	25-50 mg.
Vitamin B-12	5-25 mcg.	10-100 mcg.
Folic acid	100-400 mcg.	100-800 mcg.
Biotin	15-75 mg.	100-300 mcg.
Choline	5-25 mg.	100 mg.
Inositol	5-25 mg.	100 mg.
Bioflavonoids	5-100 mg.	100-500 mg.
PABA	2-12 mg.	15-50 mg.
Calcium	200-500 mg.	500-1,000 mg.
Magnesium	100-300 mg.	500-1,000 mg.
Iron	1-6 mg.	12-18 mg.
Copper	0.25 - 0.5 mg.	1-2 mg.
Manganese	2-10 mg.	5-25 mg.
Zinc	2-25 mg.	15-50 mg.
Chromium	10-50 mcg.	100-200 mcg.
Selenium	10-50 mcg.	100-200 mcg.
Iodine	5-60 mcg.	100-150 mcg.
Molybdenum	2-25 mcg.	50-100 mcg.
Vanadium	0-5 mcg.	0-25 mcg.

Handwritten annotations: Magnesium /00 MG; Zinc /0 M0; Chromium 50 MG; Selenium 75 M CG; Iodine 75 MG0

Handwritten note:
AMINO ACIDS
L - GLUTAMINE
L - CYSTEINE   500 MG

The formula you choose should contain the substances listed in approximately the quantities (strengths) suggested.

A Good Multiple Vitamin & Mineral Formula

Note: Nutritional needs vary among individuals according to age. Pregnant women need twice as much folic acid (800 mcg.) as most people. Menopausal or amenstrual women often need less iron than women or girls who are still menstruating. Requirements for calcium, magnesium and vitamin B-12 tend to increase in individuals of both sexes over 60. Allergic individuals usually need more manganese than others.

Children's requirements usually vary in proportion to their weight. A 60-pound child will generally need twice the nutrients of those required by a 30-pound child. Individual variability can be striking even within the same family.

For more information, see the Nutrition section of the Bibliography.

LINSEED OIL 2000 MG 2X DAY
SI BERIAN GINSENG 15-20 DROPS

APPENDIX E
FOODS POTENTIALLY HIGH IN SULFITES

These may be of concern to asthmatics.

Apples dried with preservatives	Golden raisins
Apricots dried with preservatives	Sauerkraut
Beer	Sausages
Champagne	Frozen potato products
Cheese spreads	Shellfish
Cider with preservatives	Commercial soft drinks
Cordials	Commercial juice blends
Salad bars, fresh fruit	Yogurt with fruit and preservatives
Salad bars, some vegetables	Pickles, including pickled onions
Vegetables dried with preservatives	Wines, especially sweet wines
Frozen pizza	Instant mashed potatoes

NOTE: If dried fruit looks "fresh", moist and bright in color, it probably has preservatives.

APPENDIX F
COMMON FOODS WITH A
SUBSTANTIAL SALICYLATE CONTENT

Almonds
Granny Smith apples
Broad beans
Broccoli
Sweet fresh cherries
Fresh chicory
Instant coffee
Cucumbers

Fresh eggplant
Fresh endive
Dried Calamata figs
Fresh red grapes
Grape juice
Fresh grapefruit juice
Honey
Port
Rum
Riesling wines
Sherry
Claret
Cabernet Sauvigon
Fresh spinach

Fresh mandarin oranges
Fresh mulberries
Canned mushrooms
Canned green olives
Canned okra
Fresh and canned peaches
Fresh peanuts
Peppermint-fresh, in tea or in liquor
Sweet or hot peppers
Fresh pine nuts
Fresh pistachios
Canned plums
Dried prunes
Fresh radishes
Fresh or frozen raspberries
Fresh summer squash
Fresh strawberries
Fresh tangelos
Tomato paste or sauce
Canned water chestnuts
White Vinegar
Fresh zucchini

NOTE: A wide variety of herbs and spices are also rich in salicylates, but one would have to eat huge amounts of them to get a significant dose, such as a cup of dried herbs or two spice jars full in one sitting.

GLOSSARY

Absorption: The active receiving of nutrients into the cells and tissues of the body.

Acid: Substance that liberates hydrogen ions (H^+). See pH.

Acidosis: Disturbance in the acid-base balance of the body. There is either an accumulation of acids or an excessive loss of bicarbonates.

Acute: Sharp, severe symptoms with a rapid start and usually a short duration; opposite of chronic.

Adaptogen: Substance that helps the body face stress.

Adenoid: Lymphatic tissue found in the walls of the nasopharynx.

Adrenaline: Hormone produced by the adrenal gland. British term for epinephrine.

Alkaline: Any substance that can neutralize acids. See pH.

Alkalosis: Condition in which the body becomes excessively alkaline due to an excess of alkalies or excess loss of acid or chlorides from the blood.

Allergen: Substance that brings on symptoms of allergies.

Allergy: Excessive response of the body to a specific substance which in a nonsensitive person will in the same amount produce no effect.

Alveolar: Relating to the air cells in the lungs.

Anabolic: Building phase of metabolism.

Analgesic: Relieves pain.

Anesthesize: To take away the sensation of pain or touch.

Antagonist: Something that counteracts the action of something else.

Antibiotic: Substance that inhibits the growth of or destroys microorganisms.

Antibody: Protein substance made by the body that usually serves as a defense in the bloodstream.

Antioxidant: Substance that counteracts the negative effects of oxygen or free radicals; prevents destructive oxidation.

Assimilation: The process of absorption.

Astringent: Firms tissues and organs.

Benign: Mild characteristic of an illness; not progressive.

Bogginess: Waterlogged.

Bronchospasm: Spasm of the breathing tubes.

Bronchiole: The smaller divisions of the breathing tubes.

Candidiasis: Infection of the skin or of the mucous membranes with the Candida fungus.

Capillary: Tiny blood or lymph vessel.

Catabolic: Phase of metabolism in which elements are broken down. Digestion is a catabolic process.

Cardiac: Pertaining to the heart.

Catalyst: Substance that facilitates a chemical reaction without itself being permanently changed in the reaction. Enzymes are examples of catalysts.

Catacholamine: Hormones produced by the adrenal gland, including epinephrine and norepinephrine.

Celiac disease: Intestinal absorption problem usually related to wheat sensitivity which manifests as diarrhea, malnutrition, and low level blood calcium.

Chemotaxis: Attraction of white blood cell to an area caused by a chemical stimuli initiated by injured cells.

Chronic: A disease which is persistent and often progresses slowly; opposite of acute.

Cilia: Hairlike projection of specialized surface cells which propels mucus, pus and dust particles out.

Colitis: Inflammation of the colon, with excessive secretion of mucus. Often connected with food sensitivities.

Constriction: Narrowing of a vessel or an opening.

Contagious: Transmitted easily from one person to another.

Corticosteroid: Hormone manufactured by the outer part of the adrenal gland.

Dander: Small white flake of dead skin from the coat of various animals.

Debility: Weakness in the functions or organs of the body.

Demulcent: Gentle and soothing in action, especially to the skin and mucous membranes.

Diaphragm: Large respiratory muscle separating the abdomen from the lungs.

Dilator: Expansion of a vessel or an opening.

Edema: Water retention resulting in swelling.

Electrolyte: Vital minerals in a solution which conduct electricity; most abundantly sodium, potassium, calcium and magnesium.

Ephredrine: A substance extracted from the plant Ma Huang and having a similar action to epinephrine.

Epinephrine: Substance produced by the adrenal gland. It stimulates the heart, relaxes the bronchioles and constricts the small blood vessels among other effects.

Epithelial: Refers to the layer of cells forming the surface of the skin and of the mucous membranes.

Exhalation: Breathing out.

Expectorant: Stimulates discharge of mucus from the lungs and throat.

Exudate: Accumulation of fluid in a cavity or the passing out of pus or serum.

Free radicals: Volatile molecules that can promote cellular destruction or aging.

Fungi: Division of plantlike organisms that include molds, yeast and mushrooms.

Gastrointestinal tract: The organs from the mouth to the anus which are involved with ingestion, digestion, absorption and elimination of food.

Goblet cell: Type of cell specialized in secreting mucus.

Histamine: Inflammatory substance that is normally secreted when a tissue is injured. In hay fever, excessive histamine is secreted by irritated tissues.

Immunological: Referring to the state of being immune or protected from a disease.

Immunosuppression: Preventing the immune system from responding.

Indigenous: Native to a system or region.

Infection: Condition in which the body is being invaded by disease-causing microorganisms.

Inflammation: Tissue reaction to an injury; heat.

Inhibitor: Substance that slows or stops a reaction.

Interferon: A "Paul Revere" substance produced by a cell when it is exposed to viruses to alert other cells of the infective presence.

Intercellular: Between cells.

Intracellular: Within cells.

Kaposi sarcoma: Skin disease caused by a viral infection, usually seen in AIDS/ARC patients.

Lupus, SLE (Systemic Lupus Erythematosus): Chronic systemic disease characterized by a collagen degeneration.

Lymphatic: Pertaining to the fluid found between the cells. May also refer to the vessels themselves.

Lymphocyte: Specialized white blood cell helping to provide immunity.

Macrophage: White blood cell that eats foreign substancesin the body such as bacteria.

Malabsorption: Poor absorption of nutrients from the digestive system.

Mast cell: A cell that when it feels attacked, releases histamine, an inflammatory compound.

Mastoiditis: Inflammation of the mastoid (part of thetemporal bone located near the ear).

Middle Ear: The portion of the ear that includes the eardrum and the hearing organs (stirrup, hammer, and anvil).

Micro-flora: The bacteria, viruses and fungi located in ourintestinal tract, skin and other areas.

Mineral: Simple element of which many are essential for health. They include calcium, magnesium, selenium and chromium.

Monocyte: A large white blood cell.

M.S.G. (monosodium glutamate): A salt used in cooking to enhance flavors. Produces headache, stomachache, spaciness and disorientation in some people.

Mucus: A fluid secreted by mucous membranes which serves as a protection from the outside.

Mucous membrane: The lining of passages and cavities open to the outside (nose, sinuses, mouth, throat, lungs, digestive system, urethra, and vagina).

Mycoses: Any disease produced by a fungus. Candida, thrushand athlete's foot are examples.

Pancreas: Organ producing insulin, glucagon and digestiveenzymes. It is located near the stomach.

Parasite: An organism that lives in, on or at the expense of the host without giving any benefit back to the host.

Parasympathetic nervous system: The part of the nervous system that contributes to our relaxation and to the digestion of food.

Pesticide: Chemical used to kill insects or small animals.

pH (potential of Hydrogen): A measure of acidity or alkalinity of a substance. Neutral is 7. Acid is less than 7 (7 to 0), and alkaline is more than 7 (7 to 14).

Phagocytosis: Ingestion and destruction of bacteria and other debris in the body by specialized white blood cells, e.g., phagocytes.

Polyp: Benign or malignant tumor with a stem commonly found in vascular tissue such as nose, uterus and rectum.

Precursor: A compound that precedes the formation of another compound.

Proliferation: Rapid reproduction and division of new cells.

Prostaglandin: A naturally occuring substance that affects smooth muscle and blood vessel activity.

Protein: Complex nitrogen containing compounds which break down into amino acids.

Protozoa: A type of parasite. Includes giardia and pneumocystis carinii.

Pulmonary: Relating to the lungs.

Pyrogen: A substance that produces a fever.

Radon gas: A radioactive gas produced by the disintegration of radium which may produce cancer of the lungs.

Receptor site: A place on or in the cell that binds with hormones or other substances.

Recurrence: Return of symptoms.

Red blood cell: Carrier of oxygen and CO_2 in the blood.

Reflex (cough): A cough that occurs because of the irritation to the cough center in the brain stem.

Rejuvenation: A return to health.

Replication: The way viruses reproduce.

Resolve: Return to normal.

Resorption: Absorption of waste products out of an injured area by the body.

Reversible: That which can be changed or turned back to the original direction.

Rhinitis: Inflammation of the mucosa of the nose.

Salicylates: Any salt of salicylic acid as in aspirin or wintergreen.

Scarring: Mark left on skin or organ by the healing of a wound, sore or injury.

Secondary bacterial infection: Infection that happens after a viral or fungal infection. This occurs as a result of low immune function.

Sedative: A calming effect.

Self-limiting process: A process that will heal by itself without outside intervention.

Serous cell: Cell that secretes a thin, watery fluid.

S.L.E. (systemic lupus erythematosus): See lupus.

Spasmodic: Contraction-like.

Spontaneous: Voluntary, without any aide or without any apparent cause.

Sputum: A mixture of mucus and other materials cleared from the throat or by coughing.

Stagnant: Without any movement.

Stimulant: A substance that temporarily increases the function of an organ or the whole body.

Subacute: Between acute and chronic, somewhat acute.

Subcutaneous: Beneath the skin.

Submucosal: Beneath the mucosa.

Susceptibility: The ability to be readily affected or acted upon.

Sympathetic nervous system: The part of the nervous system that prepares us for fight or flight.

Systemic: Action that happens to the whole body instead of only one part.

T-cell: White blood cell that keeps a memory of encountered enemies and will react next time they encounter this same enemy.

Thrush: Fungal infection of the mouth and throat found especially in children and immunosuppressed individuals.

Thymus gland: Gland located under the breastbone (sternum) and which supports the body's immune function.

Thyroid gland: Gland located in the front of the neck that regulates the metabolism of the body.

Toxic: Poisonous.

Trachea: Tube that brings the air from the throat to the lungs.

Upper respiratory tract: Includes the sinuses, nose, pharynx and mouth.

Vagus nerve: Nerve vital to digestion, movement and general sensory perception. Part of the parasympathic nervous sytem.

Vasoconstriction: Narrowing of the blood vessels.

Vasodilation: Expansion of the blood vessels.

Viscosity: Sticky or gummy, relating to thickness.

Vitamins: A group of complex compounds necessary for normal growth, maintenance and development of the body.

White blood cells: Colorless cells that contribute to our protection. They include lymphocytes, monocytes, macrophages, eosinophils and basophils.

HERB INDEX
COMMON NAMES TO LATIN

American Woodsgrown Ginseng	Panax quinquefolium
Astragalus	Astragalus membranaceus
Balm of Gilead	Populus candicans
Barberry	Berberis
Black Cohosh	Cimicifuga racemosa
Black Walnut (hull)	Juglans nigra
Blood Root	Sanguinaria canadensis
Boneset	Eupatorium perfoliatum
Calendula	Calendula officinalis
Cayenne	Capsicum
Cinnamon	Cinnamomum
Collinsonia	Collinsonia canadensis
Coltsfoot	Tussilago farfara
Echinacea	Echinacea angustifolia or purpurea or pallida
Elder (blossom)	Sambucus
Elecampane	Inula helenium
Eucalyptus	Eucalyptus
Eyebright	Euphrasia officinalis
Garlic	Allium sativum
Gentian	Gentiana
Ginger	Zingiber officinalis
Ginseng, Siberian	Eleutherococcus senticosus
Ginseng, Woodsgrown American	Panax quinquefolium
Grindelia	Grindelia
Hibiscus	Hibiscus
Horehound	Marrubium vulgare
Horsetail	Equisetum
Hyssop	Hyssopus officinalis
Inmortal	Asclepias asperula

Licorice	Glycyrrhiza uralensis
Lobelia	Lobelia inflata
Lungwort	Pulmonaria sticta
Ma Huang	Ephedra sinensis
Marshmallow	Althea officinalis
Mormon Tea	Ephedra viridis
Mullein	Verbascum thapsus
Myrrh	Commiphora myrrha
Nettles	Urtica dioica
Oats	Avena sativa
Ocotillo	Fouqueria splendens
Osha	Ligusticum porteri
Passion Flower	Passiflora incarnata
Pau D'Arco	Tabebuia impetiginosa
Plantain	Plantago major
Pleurisy Root	Asclepias tuberosa
Poke Root	Phytolacca decandra
Propolis	Propolis
Psyllium	Plantago ovata or psyllium
Quassia	Picraena
Red Root	Ceanothus
Siberian Ginseng	Eleutherococcus senticosus
Spikenard	Aralia racemosa
Stillingia	Stillingia sylvatica
Thuja	Thuja occidentalis
Toadflax	Linaria
Virginia Snakeroot	Aristolochia serpentaria
White Pine Bark	Pinus strobus
Wild Cherry Bark	Prunus serotina
Wild Indigo	Baptisia
Wild Oats	Avena sativa
Woodsgrown American Ginseng	Panax quinquefolium
Yarrow	Achillea millefolium
Yerba Mansa	Anemopsis
Yerba Santa	Eriodictyon

HERB INDEX
LATIN TO COMMON NAMES

Achillea millefolium	Yarrow
Allium sativum	Garlic
Althaea officinalis	Marshmallow
Anemopsis	Yerba Mansa
Aralia racemosa	Spikenard
Asclepias asperula	Inmortal
Asclepias tuberosa	Pleurisy Root
Astragalus membranaceus	Astragalus
Avena sativa	Oats or Wild Oats
Baptisia	Wild Indigo Root
Berberis	Barberry
Calendula officinalis	Calendula
Capsicum	Cayenne
Ceanothus	Red Root
Cimicifuga	Black Cohosh
Cinnamomum	Cinnamon
Collinsonia	Collinsonia or Stone Root
Commiphora myrrha	Myrrh
Echinacea angustifolia, purpurea or pallida	Echinacea, purple cone flower
Eleutherococcus senticosus	Siberian Ginseng
Ephedra sinensis	Ma Huang
Ephedra viridis	Mormon Tea
Equisetum arvensis	Horsetail
Eriodictyon	Yerba Santa
Eucalyptus	Eucalyptus
Eupatorium perfoliatum	Boneset
Euphrasia officinalis	Eyebright
Fouqueria splendens	Ocotillo
Gentiana	Gentian
Glycyrrhiza uralensis	Licorice
Grindelia	Grindelia
Hibiscus	Hibiscus

Hyssopus officinalis	Hyssop
Inula helenium	Elecampane
Juglans nigra	Black Walnut (Hull)
Ligusticum porteri	Osha
Linaria	Toadflax
Lobelia inflata	Lobelia
Marrubium vulgare	Horehound
Panax quinquefolium	Ginseng, Woodsgrown American
Passiflora incarnata	Passion Flower
Phytolacca decandra	Poke Root
Picraena	Quassia
Pinus strobus	White Pine Bark
Plantago major	Plantain
Plantago ovata or psyllium	Psyllium
Populus candicans	Balm of Gilead
Propolis	Propolis
Prunus serotina	Wild Cherry Bark
Pulmonaria sticta	Lungwort
Sambuscus	Elder (Blossom)
Sanguinaria canadensis	Bloodroot
Serpentaria	Virginia Snakeroot
Stillingia sylvatica	Stillingia
Tabebuia impetiginosa	Pau D'Arco
Thuja occidentalis	Thuja or Eastern Cedar
Tussilago farfara	Coltsfoot
Urtica dioica	Nettles
Verbascum thapsus	Mullein
Zingiber	Ginger

INDEX

Lower rib expansion, 129-130
Broccoli, 62, 83, 105, 132, 133, 136, 137, 138, 140, 149
Bronchial dilator, 5, 63, 70, 77, 90, 96, 97, 98, 120, 123
Bronchioles, 63, 93, 95
Bronchitis, 47, 102
   Acute, 67-73
   Chronic, 74, 87-91
   Infectious, 67
   Irritative, 67
Bronchospasms, 77, 93, 97
Broth (see also Healing Broth), 49, 55, 69
Brussels sprouts, 105, 135, 137, 139
Buckwheat, 89, 105, 134, 136, 138, 142
Bulgur, 135
Butter, 88, 105, 133
Buttermilk, 140

C
Cabbage, 136, 137, 139
Cadmium, 78, 79, 84
Caffeic acid glycosides, 29, 70
Caffeine (see also coffee), 5, 27, 117
Calcium, 30, 31, 72, 95, 108, 109, 122, 146
   Chart, 140
Calendula, 20, 22
Candida albicans, 40, 77, 103, 106, 107, 109
Cancer, 79, 88, 113, 116
Cantaloupe, 76, 83, 105, 133, 135, 137, 138
Caprylic acid, 51, 107, 108
Carbohydrates, 106
Carbon dioxide, 87

Carrot juice, 36, 46, 69, 113, 122, 133
Carrots, 27, 36, 62, 69, 76, 83, 95, 132, 139
Cashews, 105, 136, 142, 143
Cauliflower, 137, 139
Cayenne, 20, 22, 28, 30, 42, 43
Celery, 132
Celiac disease, 88
Cell membranes, 109
Champagne, 148
Chard, 133, 142
Cheese, 72, 88, 95, 105
   Blue, 105
   Cottage, 106, 136, 140
   Ricotta, 122, 140
   Spreads, 148
   Swiss, 140, 144
Chemical sensitivity, 71, 92, 105
Chemotaxis, 63
Cherries, 138, 149
Chestnuts, 134
Chicken, 27, 95, 134, 134
   Hearts, 144
   Liver, 133, 135, 136, 141, 143
   Noodle soup, 55
Chicory, 149
Chili peppers, 49, 149
   Green, 142
   Red, 133, 136, 137, 142
Chills, 17, 53, 59, 67
Chlorophyll, 62, 63, 76, 77
Chocolate, 37, 95, 142
Cholesterol, 107, 122
Choline, 146
Chromium, 7, 117, 146
Chronic conditions, 4, 41, 45, 74, 87

Chronic Obstructive Pulmonary Disease (C.O.P.D.), 74-79, 128
Cilia, 63, 77, 87, 97, 120, 123
Cinnamon, 21, 37, 38
Circulation (see also lung), 22, 43, 50
  Peripheral, 30
  in Throat, 44
Citrus, 138
Clay poultice, 58
Cocaine, 117
Coconut, 108
  Milk, 89, 141
Cod, 143
Cod-liver oil, 133, 139
Coffee (see also caffeine), 19, 113
  Instant, 149
Codeine, 68
Cold cuts, 105
Cold packs, 18
Colds, 17-24, 34, 53, 61
Collards, 76, 137, 140
Collinsonia, 43, 44
Colon, 67
Coltsfoot, 29, 30, 56, 76, 77, 96, 97, 101
Confusion, 18, 26
Congestion, 16, 21, 43, 102
Connective tissue, 57
Constipation, 119, 124
Copper, 45, 146
Cordials, 138
Corn, 69, 89, 105, 134
  Oil, 139
Cough, 47-52
  Chronic, 80, 87, 102
  Dry, 16, 46, 47, 67, 68, 70, 97, 111
  Productive, 16, 47, 67, 68, 87

to Relieve, 21, 50, 51, 77, 90, 124
as Symptom, 17, 25, 41, 47, 59, 67, 74, 92
Counseling, 121
Crab, 133
Cranberries, 19
Craniol-sacral work, 26
Creativity, 26
Cromolyn, 101
Cross-linkage, 124
Cucumber, 149
Cumin, 141
Currants, 139
  Black, 138
Curries, 49

D

Dairy foods, 19, 27, 37, 49, 55, 69, 83, 88, 113
Damp weather, 102
Dandelion greens, 133, 137, 140, 141, 142
Decongestants, 32, 38, 51
Demulcent (soothing), 44
Depression, 27, 88, 103
Dermatitis, 27
Diabetic acidosis, 102
Diaphoretic, 114
Diaphragm, 47, 85, 97, 128
Diarrhea, 8, 25, 34, 38
Digestive juices, 119, 124
Digitalis, 8
Diphtheria, 47
Drugs, 27, 93, 115
  Immunosuppressive, 61, 104, 109, 111
Dryness, 9
Dulse, 140, 141
Dust, 67

Whey, 88, 134
Whistling, 84
White blood cells (see also lym-
   phocytes), 18, 22, 23, 50, 57,
   61, 63, 64, 65, 70, 71, 78, 106,
   109, 113, 115
   Illustration, 60
White pine bark, 49, 50
Whooping cough, 47, 51
Wild cherry bark, 49, 50
Wild indigo, 114, 115
Wind instruments, 84
Wine, 69, 148, 149
Wrinkles, 124

Y
Yams, 83
Yarrow, 20, 21
Yeast, 83, 95
   Active, 136

   Brewer's, 134, 135, 136,
      136
   Torula, 137
Yeast infection (see also candida
   albicans) 51
Yerba mansa, 28, 29, 44, 70,
   106, 107
Yerba santa, 28, 29, 37, 76, 77
Yogurt, 88, 106, 122, 137, 140,
   148

Z
Zinc, 7, 22, 23, 28, 31, 38, 45,
   51, 57, 64, 71, 72, 78, 79, 95,
   107, 108, 115, 116, 124, 125,
   132, 146
   Chart, 144
Zucchini, 149

BIBLIOGRAPHY

HERBAL TEXTS

Bensky, Dan and Gamble, Andrew, *Chinese Herbal Medicine, Materia Medica,* Eastland Press, Seattle, WA, 1986. Gives both a Chinese medicine and pharmaceutical/clinical research overview of Chinese herbs.

Bezanger-Beauquesne, L., Pinkas, M., Torck, M., *Les Plantes dans la therapeutique moderne,* Editeur Maloine, Paris, France, 1986.
Good technical reference book on botanicals.

Clarke, J. H., *Dictionary of Materia Medica,* Third Edition, Health Science Press, Saffron Walden, Essex, U.K., 1982.
The best homeopathic materia medica available. This 3 volume set gives a complete picture of the plant's action on the body and emotions.

Curtin, L.S.M., *Healing Herbs of the Upper Rio Grande, Southwest Museum,* Los Angeles, CA, 1965.
An accurate anthropological picture of herb usage in the Southwest in the 1930's. Covers herbs such as Osha, Inmortal and Grindelia.

Der Marderosian, Ara, and Liberti, Lawrence, *Natural Produce Medicine,* George F. Stickley Co., Philadelphia, PA, 1988.
Contains a series of monographs on natural products used or claimed to be used as medicine.

Ellingwood, Finley, *American Materia Medica, Therapeutics and Pharmacology,* Eclectic Medical Publications, Portland, OR, 1983. (First published in 1898.)
A must for any serious herbalist's library. Gives a good physicological overview of plant's actions.

Felter, Harvey, Lloyd, John Uri, *King's American Dispensatory,* Eclectic Medical Publiations, Portland, OR, 1983. (First published 1922.)
As a two-volume set, this book is certainly one of the most useful in furthering in-depth herb studies.

Felter, Harvey, *The Eclectic Materia Medical, Pharmacology and Therapeutics,* Eclectic Medical Publications, Portland, OR, 1983. (First published in 1890.)
Invaluable. A little easier to use than Felter and Lloyd because the herbs are listed in alphabetical order. Excellent physiological action of each herb.

Grieve, Maude, *A Modern Herbal,* Dover Publications, New York, NY, 1971.
Written in the late 1920's, this was the first serious British herbal text for the lay person. Comprehensive 2-volume set.

Hoffman, David. *The Holistic Herbal,* The Findhorn Press, Moray, Scotland, 1983.
This is it, herbal afficionados! Highly recommended. It covers the different body systems and gives pertinent accurate information on how to use herbs responsibly.

Hutchens, Alma, *Indian Herbology of North America,* Merco, Windsor, Ontario, Canada, 1973.
An excellent book for the layman. Describes in easy to understand language how and when to use each plant.

Lecler, Henri, *Precis de phytotherapie*, Masson, Paris, France, 1976.
This book covers numerous well-documented French botanical experiments.

Moore, Michael, *Medicinal Plants of the Mountain West*, Museum of New Mexico Press, Santa Fe, NM, 1979.
An authoritative text on Southwestern plants. His physiological understanding of herbs is outstanding, his sense of humor refreshing.

Mowrey, Daniel, *The Scientific Validation of Herbal Medicine*, Cormorant Books, Utah, 1986.
Excellent references, well-documented.

Paris, R.R. and Moyse, H., *Matiere medicale*, Masson and Cie, Paris, France, 1967.
Offers a pharmacopia overview of French medicinal plants.

Ross, M.S.F., and Brain, K.R., *An introduction to Phytopharmacy*, Pitman Medical Publishing Co., Ltd., Kent, U.K., 1977.
Gives a medical phyto-chemical overview of plants used in the United Kingdom.

Schauenberg, Paul, and Paris, Ferdinand, *Guide to Medicinal Plants*, Keats Publishing, New Canaan, CT, 1977.
Divides plants according to their chemical constituents.

Santillo, Humbart, *Natural Healing with Herbs*, Hohm Press, Prescott Valley, AZ, 1984.
Useful herb book for the layman. Covers a good number of plants and their usage.

Tyler, Varro, Brady, Lymon; Robbers, James, *Pharmacognosy*, Eighth Edition, Lea and Febiger, Philadelphia, PA, 1981.
Introduces and discusses plants still used in pharmacy today.

Valnet, Jean, *Phytotherapie*, 2nd edition, Librairie Maloine, Paris, France, 1976.
A great book on French herbal medicine, very thorough and complete.

Valnet, Jean, *Aromatherapie*, 8th edition, Maloine, Paris, France. 1976.
One of the best books on oil utilization in modern medicine. Quite technical.

Wager, H., Bladt, S.; and Zgainski, E.M., *Plant Drug Analysis*, Springer Verlag, New York, NY, 1983.
One of the definitive texts on plant identification utilizing Thin Layer Chromatography.

Weiss, Rudolf F., *Herbal Medicine,* Beaconsfield/Arcanum, Beaconsfield, England, 1988.
An absolute must for any herbal practitioner or any professional wanting to understand and utilize botanicals in his practice.

Propolis Apimondia Publishing House, Bucharest, 1978.
A compilation of clinical use of propolis. Impressive.

SPECIALIZED RESPIRATORY TEXTS

Burrows, Benjamin; Knudson, Ronald; Quan, Stuart and Kettel, Louis, *Respiratory Disorders, Year Book Medical Publications*, Chicago, 1983.

Dewey, Jackie, *Of Life and Breath*, Warner Books, New York, NY, 1986.

Flint, K.C., *Bronchoalveolar Mast Cells and Asthma*, Springer Verlag, London, 1987.

Lehnert, Bruce and Schackter, Ned, *The Pharmacology of Respiratory Care*, The C.V. Mosby Co., St. Louis, KS, 1980.

Netter, Frank H., *Respiratory System, The Ciba Collection of Medical Illustrations*, Volume 7, Summit, N.J. 1979.

Murray, John, *The Normal Lung*, W. B. Saunders Co., Philadelphia, PA, 1986.

Plowman, P.N., *Respiratory Medicine*, Medical Examination Publishing Co., New York, NY, 1987.

Rau, Joseph, *Respiratory Therapy Pharmacology*, Year Book Medical Publishers, Chicago, IL, 1984.

Witkowski, Arthur, *Pulmonary Assessment: A Clinical Guide*, J.B. Lippincott Co., Philadelphia, PA, 1985.

Handbook of Nonprescription Drugs, 8th Edition, American Pharmaceutical Association, The National Professional Society of Pharmacists, Washington, D.C., 1986.

EMOTIONAL SUPPORT TEXTS

Cousins, Norman, *Anatomy of an Illness*, Bantam Books, New York, NY, 1979.

Harrison, John, M.D., *Love Your Disease*, Hay House, Inc., Santa Monica, CA, 1984.

Hay, Louise, *Heal Your Body*, Hay House, Inc., Santa Monica, CA, 1988.

Hendricks, Gay and Kathleen, Ph.D., *Centering and the Art of Intimacy*, Prentice Hall Press, New York, NY, 1985.

Jampolsky, Gerald, M.D., *Love is Letting Go of Fear*, Celestial Arts, Berkeley, CA, 1979.

Keyes, Ken, *Handbook to Higher Consciousness*, Living Love Publications, St. Mary, KT, 1981.

People with AIDS Coalition, Inc., *Surviving and Thriving with AIDS: Hints for the Newly Diagnosed*, NY, 1987

Siegel, Bernie, M.D., *Love, Medicine, and Miracles*, Harper and Row, New York, NY, 1986.

Simonton, Carl and Stephanie, and Creighton, J., *Getting Well Again*, Bantam Books, New York, NY, 1980.

NUTRITION

Badgley, Lawrence, *Healing AIDS Naturally*, Human Energy Press, San Bruno, CA, 1987.

Excellent and well-researched introduction to alternative therapies for the immune system, including foods, herbs, supplements and feelings.

Ballentine, Rudolph, *Diet and Nutrition: A Holistic Approach*, Himalayan International Institute, Hanesdale, PA, 1978.

Clearest and best introduction to nutrition we know. Fascinating, readable and packed with information. Includes Western and Ayurvedic approaches.

Buist, Robert, *Food Chemical Sensitivity*, Harper & Row, Sydney, Australia, 1986.

A must for those with asthma, chronic bronchitis, or suspected sensitivities. Detailed tables of essential information.

Crook, William, *The Yeast Connection*, Professional Books, Jackson, TN, 1985.

A good text for the layperson about yeast and its role in illness. Includes specific diets.

Davies, Stephen and Stewart, Alan, *Nutritional Medicine*, Pan Books, London, 1987 (available in U.S. through Avon, 1990?).

Comprehensive coverage of nutritional self-care for the whole family.

Goodhart, Robert S. and Maurice E. Shols, eds., *Modern Nutrition in Health and Disease*, Lea & Febiger, Philadelphia, PA, 1980.

Best technical reference book available on nutrition.

Kane, Patricia, *Food Makes the Difference*, Simon & Schuster, New York, NY, 1985.

Specially designed for parents working with children with special nutritional needs. Thorough, excellent, with many recipes and a valuable section on "Easing into Rotation Diets."

Nutrition Search, Inc., *Nutrition Almanac*, McGraw Hill Book Company, New York, NY, 1979.

Good food composition tables.

Reading, Chris M. and Ross, S. Meillon, *Your Family Tree Connection*, Keats Publishing, Inc., New Canaan, CT, 1988.

A deceptively simple book which may revolutionize our approach to nutrition. Explores genetic influences on nutritional needs and sensitivities.

Roth, Geneen, *Breaking Free From Compulsive Eating*, Penguin Books, NY, 1984.

Truss, C. Orion, *The Missing Diagnosis*, The Missing Diagnosis (press), Birmingham, AL, 1982.

In-depth approach to yeast illnesses. The classic text.

OTHER

Lad, Vasant, *Ayureveda: The Science of Self-Healing*, Lotus Press, Santa Fe, NM, 1984.

Clear and simple introduction to this ancient East Indian system of healing.

Morningstar, Amadea, *The Ayurvedic Cookbook*, Lotus Press, Santa Fe, NM, 1990.

A practical and informative cookbook that shows you how to apply Ayurveda in your everyday life.

Svoboda, Robert E., Prakruti: *Your Ayurvedic Constitution*, Geocom, Albuquerque, NM, 1988.

Articulate, well-written discussion of Ayurveda for those who are interested in understanding more about this system.

DANIEL O. GAGNON has been a practicing herbalist since 1976. Canadian-born, he relocated in 1979 to Santa Fe, New Mexico, where he furthered his studies in medical herbalism, pharmacology and related subjects at the Santa Fe College of Natural Medicine, the College of Santa Fe, and the University of New Mexico's College of Pharmacy. He manufactures liquid herbal extracts that are provided to retail outlets and medical practitioners. He is also the owner of a retail botanical store, Herbs Etc.

Daniel has taught seminars in herbal therapeutics in the United States and Canada, including New York City, Miami, Atlanta, Boulder, Washington, D.C., Toronto, and Montreal, and has been on the faculty of the Institute of Traditional Medicine in Santa Fe. He has written for such publications as WHOLE FOODS, NATURAL LIFESTYLING, THE HERB MAGAZINE and NATURAL FOODS MERCHANDISER. He frequently is called upon as an herbal consultant by medical doctors, naturopaths, chiropractors and acupuncturists.

R. AMADEA MORNINGSTAR has been a practicing clinical nutritionist and teacher in Santa Fe for seventeen years. She received a B.S. in nutrition and food sciences from the University of California at Berkeley and an M.A. in counseling from Southwestern College in Santa Fe. She also pursued studies in human biology at Stanford University and nutrition at the University of Texas at Austin. She has been a member of the faculties of the Santa Fe College of Natural Medicine, the Institute of Traditional Medicine in Santa Fe, and the Ayurvedic Institute of Albuquerque, New Mexico.

During the last five years, Amadea has integrated counseling and creative expression into her private consultations with individuals, couples and families. She acts as a nutritional consultant for other practitioners, and for a wide variety of non-profit organizations. She has written THE AYURVEDIC COOKBOOK with Urmila Desai (Lotus Press, 1990).